CARDIOVASCULAR
PHYSIOLOGY

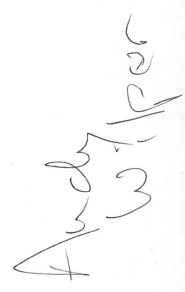

CARDIOVASCULAR PHYSIOLOGY

Fourth Edition

David E. Mohrman, Ph.D.

Associate Professor, Department of Medical and Molecular Physiology

Lois Jane Heller, Ph.D.

Professor, Department of Medical and Molecular Physiology

School of Medicine
University of Minnesota, Duluth
Duluth, Minnesota

McGraw-Hill
Health Professions Division

New York   St. Louis   San Francisco   Auckland   Bogotá   Caracas   Lisbon
London   Madrid   Mexico City   Milan   Montreal   New Delhi   San Juan
Singapore   Sydney   Tokyo   Toronto

McGraw-Hill

*A Division of The **McGraw·Hill** Companies*

CARDIOVASCULAR PHYSIOLOGY

Copyright © 1997, 1991, 1986, 1981 by *The **McGraw-Hill** Companies,* Inc. All rights reserved. Printed in the United States of America. Except as permitted under the United States Copyright Act of 1976, no part of this publication may be reproduced or distributed in any form or by any means, or stored in a data base or retrieval system, without prior written permission of the publisher.

4 5 6 7 8 9 10 DOC/DOC 0 9 8 7 6 5 4 3 2 1 0

ISBN 0-07-028025-8

This book was set in Times Roman by Digitype.
The editors were Joseph Hefta and Steven Melvin;
The production supervisor was Clare Stanley.

R. R. Donnelley and Sons, Inc., was the printer and binder.

Library of Congress Cataloging-in-Publication Data

Mohrman, David E.
    Cardiovascular physiology / David E. Mohrman, Lois Jane Heller. —
4th ed.
       p.   cm.
    Includes bibliographical references and index.
    ISBN 0-07-028025-8
    1. Cardiovascular system — Physiology.   I. Heller, Lois Jane.
II. Title.
    [DNLM: 1. Cardiovascular System — physiology.   WG 102 M699c 1996]
QP101.M56   1996
612.1 — dc20
DNLM/DLC
for Library of Congress   96-35519

CONTENTS

Appendices

PREFACE

This text is intended to provide students with the core of information and concepts necessary to develop a firm understanding of how the intact cardiovascular system operates. Specifically stated learning objectives and study questions for each chapter allow the student to test his or her mastery of the material presented. This format lends itself to independent study, which may (but need not) be supplemented by additional lecture material. References are supplied for each chapter to provide interested students with access to the pertinent research literature.

We feel strongly that cardiovascular instruction should give the student not simply a collection of facts but also an understanding of how the intact cardiovascular system operates. Cardiovascular physiology is often a student's first exposure to the operation of a complete organ system, and the student therefore often finds it confusing to deal with the continual interactions that occur among the various system components. Consequently, we have tried to direct our presentation throughout toward the overall operation of the cardiovascular system rather than attempting to present all available facts.

The changes and additions to this fourth edition are the result of several factors, including new research findings, our own experience in using the previous editions, and helpful comments and criticisms from colleagues and students. For example, we have significantly revised and expanded coverage of the cellular aspects of cardiac and smooth muscle function to reflect recent research advances in these areas. Because of the current trend in medical education toward integrated courses, the scope of the text has been broadened somewhat. For example, we have added information on blood and blood clotting. As in previous revisions, we have tried to improve the usefulness of the text from the student's perspective. That is, we strive for a readable, logically arranged text that makes the complex cardiovascular system understandable to the reader. To that end, we have done some rearranging and considerable rewriting, improved and added figures, and added study questions and appendices.

We wish to express our sincere thanks to all colleagues and students who have supplied us with suggestions for improving this text, and we will welcome your comments on and criticisms of the fourth edition.

1

HOMEOSTASIS AND CARDIOVASCULAR TRANSPORT

OBJECTIVES

The student understands the basic principles of cardiovascular transport and their roles in maintaining homeostasis:

1 Defines homeostasis.
2 Identifies the major body fluid compartments and states the approximate volume of each.
3 Describes the basic composition of the fluid and cellular portions of blood.
4 Diagrams the blood flow pathways between the heart and other major body organs.
5 Lists the two conditions, provided by the cardiovascular system, that are essential for regulating the composition of interstitial fluid.
6 States the relationship among blood flow, blood pressure, and vascular resistance.
7 Predicts the percentage change in flow through a tube caused by a doubling of tube length, tube radius, fluid viscosity, or pressure difference.
8 Defines bulk transport and diffusion and lists the factors that determine the rate of each.
9 Given data, uses the Fick principle to calculate the rate of removal of a solute from blood as it passes through an organ.
10 Describes how capillary wall permeability to a solute is related to the size and lipid solubility of the solute.
11 Lists the factors that influence transcapillary fluid movement and, given data, predicts the direction of transcapillary fluid movement.
12 Describes the lymphatic vessel system and its role in preventing fluid accumulation in the interstitial space.

HOMEOSTASIS AND THE CARDIOVASCULAR SYSTEM

A nineteenth-century French physiologist, Claude Bernard (1813–1878), first recognized that all higher organisms actively and constantly strive to prevent the external environment from upsetting the conditions necessary for life within the organism. Thus the temperature, oxygen concentration, pH, ionic composition, osmolarity, and many other important variables of our *internal environment* are closely controlled. This process of maintaining the "constancy" of our internal environment has come to be known as *homeostasis.* To accomplish this task, an elaborate material transport network, the cardiovascular system, has evolved.

Various compartments of watery fluids, known collectively as the *total body water,* account for about 60 percent of body weight. This water is distributed among the *intracellular, interstitial,* and *plasma* spaces as indicated in Fig. 1-1. About two-thirds of our body water is contained within cells and communicates with the interstitial fluid across the plasma membranes of cells. Of the fluid that is outside cells, only a small amount, the *plasma volume,* circulates within the cardiovascular system. Blood is composed of plasma and roughly an equal volume of formed elements (primarily red cells). The circulating plasma fluid communicates with the interstitial fluid across the walls of small capillary vessels.

The interstitial fluid is the immediate environment of individual cells. These cells must draw their nutrients from and release their products into the interstitial fluid. The interstitial fluid cannot, however, be considered a large reservoir for nutrients or a large sink for metabolic products since its volume is less than half that of the cells that it serves. The well-being of individual cells therefore depends heavily on the homeostatic mechanisms that regulate the composition of the interstitial fluid. This task is accomplished by continuously exposing the interstitial fluid to "fresh" circulating plasma fluid.

As the blood passes through capillaries, solutes exchange between the plasma and the interstitial fluid by the process of diffusion. The net result of

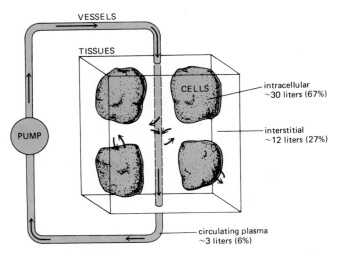

Figure 1-1 Major body fluid compartments with average volumes indicated for a 70-kg human. Total body water is about 60 percent of body weight. Numbers in parentheses indicate approximate percentage of total body water in each compartment.

transcapillary diffusion is always that the interstitial fluid tends to take on the composition of the incoming blood. If, for example, the potassium ion concentration in the interstitium of a particular skeletal muscle were higher than that in the plasma entering the muscle, potassium would diffuse into the blood as it passed through the muscle's capillaries. Since this removes potassium from the interstitial fluid, the interstitial potassium ion concentration would decrease. It would stop decreasing when net movement of potassium into capillaries no longer occurred, i.e., when the interstitial concentration reached that of the incoming plasma.

Two conditions are essential for this circulatory mechanism to effectively control the composition of interstitial fluid: (1) there must be adequate blood flow through the tissue capillaries, and (2) the chemical composition of the incoming (or arterial) blood must be controlled to be that which is desired in the interstitial fluid. These conditions are met by the design and operation of the cardiovascular system.

MAJOR COMPONENTS OF THE CARDIOVASCULAR SYSTEM
Blood

Blood is a complex fluid that serves as the medium for transporting substances between the tissues of the body and performs a host of other functions as well. Normally about 40 percent of the volume of whole blood is occupied by blood cells that are suspended in the watery fluid, *plasma,* which accounts for the rest of the volume. The fraction of blood volume occupied by cells is a clinically important parameter termed the *hematocrit:*

Hematocrit = cell volume/total blood volume

Blood Cells   Blood contains three general types of "formed elements": red cells, white cells, and platelets (see Appendix A). All are formed in bone marrow from a common stem cell. Red cells are by far the most abundant. They are specialized to carry oxygen from the lungs to other tissues by binding oxygen to *hemoglobin,* an iron-containing heme protein concentrated within red cells. Because of the presence of hemoglobin, blood can transport 40 to 50 times the amount of oxygen that plasma alone could carry. In addition, the hydrogen ion buffering capacity of hemoglobin is vitally important to the blood's capacity to transport carbon dioxide.

A small but important fraction of the cells in blood are white cells or *leukocytes.* Leukocytes are involved in immune processes. Appendix A gives more information on the types and function of leukocytes. Platelets are small cell fragments importantly involved in the blood-clotting process.

Plasma   *Plasma* is the liquid component of blood and, as indicated in Appendix B, is a complex solution of electrolytes and proteins. *Serum* is the fluid obtained from a blood sample after it has been allowed to clot. For all practical purposes, the composition of serum is identical to that of plasma except that it contains none of the clotting proteins.

Inorganic *electrolytes* (inorganic ions such as sodium, potassium, chloride, and bicarbonate) are the most concentrated solutes in plasma. Of these, sodium and chloride are by far the most abundant and, therefore, are primarily responsible for plasma's normal osmolarity of about 300 mosm/liters. To a first approximation, the "stock" of the plasma soup is a 150 mM solution of sodium chloride. Such a solution is called isotonic saline and has many clinical uses as a fluid that is compatible with cells.

Plasma normally contains many different *proteins.* Most plasma proteins can be classified as either *albumins, globulins,* or *fibrinogen* on the basis of different physical and chemical characteristics used to separate them. More than 100 distinct plasma proteins have been identified and each presumably serves some specific function. Many plasma proteins are involved in blood clotting or immune/defense reactions. Many others are important carrier proteins for a variety of substances including fatty acids, iron, copper, vitamin D, and certain hormones.

Proteins do not readily cross capillary walls and, in general, their plasma concentrations are much higher than their concentrations in the interstitial fluid. As will be discussed later in this chapter, plasma proteins play an important osmotic role in transcapillary fluid movement and thus the distribution of extracellular volume between the blood and interstitial compartment. *Albumin* plays an especially strong role in this regard simply because it is by far the most abundant of the plasma proteins.

Plasma also serves as the vehicle for transporting nutrients and waste products. Thus a plasma sample contains many small organic molecules such as glucose, amino acids, urea, creatinine, and uric acid whose measured values are useful in clinical diagnosis.

Heart and Vessels

The overall functional arrangement of the cardiovascular system is illustrated in Fig. 1-2. Since a functional rather than an anatomic viewpoint is expressed in this figure, the heart appears in three places: as the right heart pump, as the left heart pump, and as the heart muscle tissue. It is common practice to view the cardiovascular system as (1) the *pulmonary circulation,* composed of the right heart pump and the lungs, and (2) the *systemic circulation,* in which the left heart pump supplies blood to the systemic organs (all structures except the gas exchange portion of the lungs). The pulmonary and systemic circulations are arranged in series, i.e., one after the other. Consequently, the right and left hearts must pump an identical volume of blood each minute. This amount is called the *cardiac output.* A cardiac output of 5 to 6 liters/min is normal for a resting individual.

As indicated in Fig. 1-2, the systemic organs are functionally arranged in parallel (i.e., side by side) within the cardiovascular system. There are two important consequences of this parallel arrangement. First, nearly all systemic or-

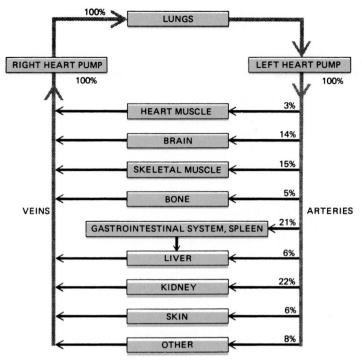

Figure 1-2 Cardiovascular circuitry indicating the percentage distribution of cardiac output to various organ systems in a resting individual.

gans receive blood of identical composition—that which has just left the lungs and is known as *arterial blood.* Second, the flow through any one of the systemic organs can be controlled independently of the flow through the other organs. Thus, for example, the cardiovascular response to whole body exercise can involve increased blood flow through some organs, decreased blood flow through others, and unchanged blood flow through yet others.

Many of the organs in the body help perform the task of continually reconditioning the blood circulating in the cardiovascular system. Key roles are played by organs such as the lungs, which communicate with the external environment. As is evident from the arrangement shown in Fig. 1-2, any blood that has just passed through a systemic organ returns to the right heart and is pumped through the lungs, where oxygen and carbon dioxide are exchanged. Thus the blood's gas composition is always reconditioned immediately after leaving a systemic organ.

Like the lungs, many of the systemic organs also serve to recondition the composition of blood, although the flow circuitry precludes their doing so each time the blood completes one circuit. The kidneys, for example, continually adjust the electrolyte composition of the blood passing through them. Because the blood conditioned by the kidneys mixes freely with all the circulating blood and because electrolytes and water freely pass through most capillary walls, the kidneys control the electrolyte balance of the entire internal environment. To achieve this, it is necessary that a given unit of blood pass often through the kidneys. In fact, the kidneys (under resting conditions) normally receive about one-fourth of the cardiac output. This greatly exceeds the amount of flow that is necessary to supply the nutrient needs of the renal tissue. This situation is common to organs that have a blood-conditioning function.

Blood-conditioning organs can also withstand, at least temporarily, severe reductions of blood flow. Skin, for example, can easily tolerate a large reduction in blood flow when it is necessary to conserve body heat. Most of the large abdominal organs also fall into this category. The reason is simply that because of their blood-conditioning functions, their normal blood flow is far in excess of that necessary to maintain their basal metabolic needs.

The brain, heart muscle, and skeletal muscles typify organs in which blood flows solely to supply the metabolic needs of the tissue. They do not recondition blood for the benefit of any other organ. Flow to brain and heart muscle is normally only slightly greater than that required for their metabolism, and they do not tolerate blood flow interruptions well. Unconsciousness can occur within a few seconds after stoppage of cerebral flow, and permanent brain damage can occur in as little as 4 min without flow. Similarly, the heart muscle (myocardium) normally consumes about 75 percent of the oxygen supplied to it, and the heart's pumping ability begins to deteriorate within beats of a coronary flow interruption. As we shall see later, the task of providing adequate blood flow to the brain and the heart muscle receives a high priority in the overall operation of the cardiovascular system.

BASIC PHYSICS OF CARDIOVASCULAR TRANSPORT

The cardiovascular system is a network for moving substances from one location in the body to another. Its efficient design permits it to use a very limited volume of circulating fluid to control the chemical composition of the entire internal environment. The operation utilizes only the processes of fluid flow and diffusion and thus an understanding of the simple physical principles which govern these processes is fundamental to understanding all cardiovascular function.

The Basic Flow Equations

One of the most important keys to comprehending how the cardiovascular system operates is a thorough understanding of the relationship among the physical factors that determine the rate of fluid flow through a tube.

The tube depicted in Fig. 1-3 represents a segment of any vessel in the body. It has a certain length (L) and a certain internal radius (r) through which blood flows. Fluid flows through the tube only when the pressures in the fluid at

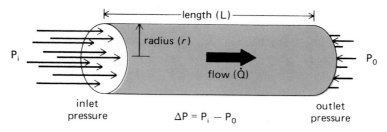

Figure 1-3 Factors influencing flow through a tube.

the inlet and outlet ends (P_i and P_o) are unequal, i.e., when there is a pressure difference (ΔP) between the ends. Pressure differences supply the driving force for flow. Because friction develops between moving fluid and the stationary walls of a tube, vessels tend to resist fluid movement through them. This *vascular resistance* is a measure of how difficult it is to make fluid flow through the tube, i.e., how much of a pressure difference it takes to cause a certain flow. The all-important relation among flow, pressure difference, and resistance is described by the *basic flow equation* as follows:

$$\text{Flow} = \frac{\text{pressure difference}}{\text{resistance}}$$

$$\dot{Q} = \frac{\Delta P}{R}$$

where $\dot{Q}$ = flow rate (volume/time)
  ΔP = pressure difference (mmHg[1])
  R = resistance to flow (mmHg × time/volume)

The basic flow equation may be applied not only to a single tube but to complex networks of tubes, e.g., to the vascular bed of an organ or to the entire systemic system. The flow through the brain, for example, is determined by the difference in pressure between cerebral arteries and veins divided by the overall resistance to flow through the vessels in the cerebral vascular bed. It should be evident from the basic flow equation that there are only two ways in which blood flow through any organ can be changed: (1) by changing the pressure difference across its vascular bed, or (2) by changing its vascular resistance. Most often, it is changes in an organ's vascular resistance that cause the flow through the organ to change.

---

[1] Although pressure is most correctly expressed in units of force per unit area, it is customary to express pressures within the cardiovascular system in millimeters of mercury. For example, mean arterial pressure may be said to be 100 mmHg because it is the same as the pressure existing at the bottom of a mercury column 100 mm high. All cardiovascular pressures are expressed relative to atmospheric pressure, which is approximately 760 mmHg.

From the work of the French physician Jean Leonard Marie Poiseuille (1799–1869), who performed experiments on fluid flow through small glass capillary tubes, we know that the resistance to flow through a cylindrical tube depends on several factors including the radius and length of the tube and the viscosity of the fluid flowing through it. These factors influence resistance to flow as follows:

$$R = \frac{8L\eta}{\pi r^4}$$

where r = inside radius of the tube
L = tube length
η = fluid viscosity

Note that the internal radius of the tube is raised to the fourth power in this equation. Thus even small changes in the internal radius of a tube have a very large influence on its resistance to flow. For example, halving the inside radius of a tube will increase its resistance to flow by 16-fold.

The preceding equations may be combined into one expression known as the *Poiseuille equation*, which includes all the terms that influence flow through a cylindrical vessel.[2]

$$\dot{Q} = \Delta P \frac{\pi r^4}{8L\eta}$$

Again note that flow occurs only when a pressure difference exists. It is not surprising then that arterial blood pressure is an extremely important and carefully regulated cardiovascular variable. Also note once again that, for any given pressure difference, tube radius has a very large influence on the flow through a tube. It is logical, therefore, that organ blood flows are regulated primarily through changes in the radius of vessels within organs. Whereas vessel length and blood viscosity are factors that influence vascular resistance, they are not variables which can be easily manipulated for the purpose of moment-to-moment control of blood flow.

Bulk Transport and the Fick Principle

Substances are carried between organs within the cardiovascular system by the process of *bulk transport*, the simple process of being swept along with the flow of the fluid in which they are contained. The rate at which a substance (X) is transported by this process depends solely on the concentration of the substance in the blood and the blood flow rate.

---

[2] Poiseuille's equation properly applies only to a homogeneous fluid flowing through rigid nontapered tubes with a certain flow pattern called *laminar flow*. Although not all these conditions are rigidly met for any vessel within the body, the approximation is close enough to permit general conclusions to be drawn from Poiseuille's equation.

Transport rate = flow rate × concentration

or

$$\dot{X} = \dot{Q}[X]$$

where $\dot{X}$ = rate of transport of X (mass/time)
$\dot{Q}$ = blood flow rate (volume/time)
[X] = concentration of X in blood (mass/volume)

It is evident from the preceding equation that only two means are available for altering the rate at which a substance is carried to an organ: (1) a change in the blood flow rate through the organ or (2) a change in the arterial blood concentration of the substance. The preceding equation might be used, for example, to calculate how much oxygen is carried to a certain skeletal muscle each minute. Note, however, that this calculation would not indicate whether the muscle actually used the oxygen carried to it.

One can extend the bulk transport principle to determine a tissue's rate of utilization of a substance by simultaneously considering the transport rate of the substance to *and from* the tissue. The relationship that results is referred to as the *Fick principle* (Adolf Fick, a German physician, 1829–1901) and may be formally stated as follows:

$$\dot{X}_{tc} = \dot{Q}([X]_a - [X]_v)$$

where $\dot{X}_{tc}$ = transcapillary efflux rate of X (mass/time)
$\dot{Q}$ = blood flow rate (volume/time)
$[X]_{a,v}$ = arterial and venous concentrations of X

The Fick principle essentially says that the amount of a substance that goes into an organ in a given period of time ($\dot{Q}[X]_a$) minus the amount that comes out ($\dot{Q}[X]_v$) must equal the tissue utilization rate of that substance.

Transcapillary Solute Diffusion

Capillaries act as efficient exchange sites where most substances cross the capillary walls simply by *passively diffusing* from regions of high concentration to regions of low concentration.[3] As in any diffusion problem, there are four factors that determine the diffusion rate of a substance between the blood and the interstitial fluid: (1) the concentration difference, (2) the surface area for exchange, (3) the diffusion distance, and (4) the permeability of the capillary wall to the diffusing substance.[4]

---

[3] Evidence indicates that the capillary endothelial cells can metabolize or produce certain substances. In these special cases, the capillary wall cannot be considered as a passive barrier between the intravascular and interstitial compartments.

[4] These factors are combined in an equation (Fick's first law of diffusion) which describes the rate of diffusion ($\dot{X}_d$) of a substance X across a barrier: $\dot{X}_d = DA\,\Delta[X]/\Delta L$, where D, A, $\Delta[X]$, and ΔL represent the diffusion coefficient, surface area, concentration difference, and diffusion distance, respectively.

Capillary beds allow huge amounts of materials to enter and leave blood because they maximize the area across which exchange can occur while minimizing the distance over which the diffusing substances must travel. Capillaries are extremely fine vessels with a *lumen* (inside) diameter of about 5 μm, a wall thickness of approximately 1 μm, and an average length of perhaps 0.5 mm. (For comparison, a human hair is roughly 100 μm in diameter.) Capillaries are distributed in incredible numbers in organs and communicate intimately with all regions of the interstitial space. It is estimated, for example, that a single cubic centimeter of heart muscle contains about 2,000,000 individual capillaries with a total surface area for transcapillary diffusional exchange of about 400 cm^2. This is roughly the surface area of this page. The interstitial volume of a cubic centimeter of tissue, if spread over this page, would form a layer only about 8 μm thick. Diffusion is a tremendously powerful mechanism for material exchange when operating over such a short distance and through such a large area. We are far from being able to duplicate—in an artificial lung or kidney, for example—the favorable geometry for diffusional exchange which exists in our own tissues.

As diagrammed in Fig. 1-4, the capillary wall itself consists of only a single thickness of endothelial cells joined to form a tube. The ease with which a particular solute crosses the capillary wall is expressed in a parameter called its capillary *permeability*. Permeability takes into account all the factors (diffusion coefficient, diffusion distance, and surface area), except concentration difference, that affect the rate at which a solute crosses the capillary wall.

Careful experimental studies on how rapidly different substances cross capillary walls indicate that two fundamentally distinct pathways exist for transcapillary exchange. Lipid-soluble substances, such as the gases oxygen and carbon dioxide, cross the capillary wall easily. Since the lipid endothelial cell plasma membranes are not a significant diffusion barrier for lipid-soluble substances, transcapillary movement of these substances can occur through the entire capillary surface area.

The capillary permeability to small polar particles such as sodium and potassium ions is about 10,000-fold less than it is to oxygen. Nevertheless, the capillary permeability to small ions is several orders of magnitude higher than the permeability that would be expected if the ions were forced to move through the lipid plasma membranes. It is therefore postulated that capillaries are somehow perforated at intervals with water-filled channels or *pores*.[5] Calculations from diffusion data indicate that the collective cross-sectional area of the pores relative to the total capillary surface area varies greatly between capillaries in different organs. Brain capillaries appear to be very tight (have few pores), whereas capillaries in the kidney and fluid-producing glands are much more leaky. On the average, however, pores constitute only a very small fraction of total capillary surface area—perhaps 0.01 percent. This area is, nevertheless, sufficient to allow very rapid equilibration of small water-soluble substances between the plasma and interstitial fluids of most organs. Thus the concentrations

---

[5]   Pores, as such, are not readily apparent in electron micrographs of capillary endothelial cells. Most believe the pores are really clefts in the junctions between endothelial cells.

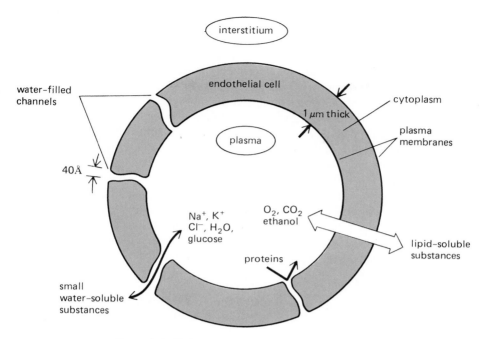

Figure 1-4   Pathways for transcapillary solute diffusion.

of inorganic ions measured in a plasma sample can be taken to indicate their concentrations throughout the entire extracellular space.

An effective maximum diameter of about 40 Å has been assigned to individual pores since substances with molecular diameters larger than this essentially do not cross capillary walls.[6] Thus albumin and other proteins in the plasma are normally confined to the plasma space.[7]

Transcapillary Fluid Movement

In addition to providing a diffusion pathway for polar molecules, the water-filled channels that traverse capillary walls permit fluid flow through the capillary wall. Net shifts of fluid between the capillary and interstitial compartments are important for a host of physiological functions, including the maintenance of circulating blood volume, intestinal fluid absorption, tissue edema formation, and saliva, sweat, and urine production. Net fluid movement out of capillaries is

---

[6]   The precise mechanism responsible for this size-selectivity remains controversial. It may stem from the actual physical dimensions of the "pores," or it may represent the filtering properties of a fiber matrix that either covers or fills the pores.

[7]   In reality, macromolecules do cross capillary walls ever so slowly by a pinocytotic mechanism sometimes referred to as the "large pore" system. Even with this special system, the capillary protein permeability is still about 1000-fold less than either sodium or glucose permeability.

referred to as *filtration,* and fluid movement into capillaries is called *reabsorption.*

Fluid flows through transcapillary channels in response to pressure differences between the interstitial and intracapillary fluids according to the basic flow equation. However, both *hydrostatic* and *osmotic pressures* influence transcapillary fluid movement. We have discussed previously how hydrostatic pressure provides the driving force for causing blood flow along vessels. The hydrostatic pressure inside capillaries, P_c, is about 25 mmHg and is the driving force which causes blood to return to the right heart from the capillaries of systemic organs. In addition, however, the 25-mmHg hydrostatic intracapillary pressure tends to cause fluid to flow through the transcapillary pores into the interstitium where the hydrostatic pressure (P_i) is near 0 mmHg. Thus, there is normally a large hydrostatic pressure difference favoring fluid filtration across the capillary wall. Our entire plasma volume would soon be in the interstitium if there were not some counteracting force tending to draw fluid into the capillaries. The balancing force is an osmotic pressure that arises from the fact that plasma has a higher protein concentration than does interstitial fluid.

Recall that solvent always tends to move from regions of low to regions of high total solute concentration in establishing osmotic equilibrium. Also recall that osmotic forces are quantitatively expressed in terms of osmotic pressure; the osmotic pressure of a given solution is defined as the hydrostatic pressure necessary to prevent osmotic water movement into the test solution when it is exposed to pure water across a membrane permeable only to water. The total osmotic pressure of a solution is proportional to the total number of solute particles in the solution. Plasma, for example, has a total osmotic pressure of about 5000 mmHg—nearly all of which is attributable to dissolved mineral salts such as NaCl and KCl. As discussed, the capillary permeability to small ions is quite high. Their concentrations in plasma and interstitial fluid are very nearly equal and, consequently, they do not affect transcapillary fluid movement. There is, however, a small but important difference in the osmotic pressures of plasma and interstitial fluid which is due to the presence of albumin and other proteins in the plasma which are normally absent from the interstitial fluid. A special term, *oncotic pressure,* is used to denote that portion of a fluid's osmotic pressure which is due to particles which do not move freely across capillaries. Because of the plasma proteins, the oncotic pressure of plasma (π_c) is about 25 mmHg. Due to the absence of proteins, the oncotic pressure of the interstitial fluid (π_i) is near 0 mmHg. Thus there is normally a large osmotic force for fluid reabsorption into capillaries. The forces which influence transcapillary fluid movement are summarized on the left side of Fig. 1-5.

The relationship among the factors that influence transcapillary fluid movement, known as the *Starling hypothesis,*[8] can be expressed by the equation:

$$\text{Net filtration rate} = K[(P_c - P_i) - (\pi_c - \pi_i)]$$

[8]   After the British physiologist Ernest Starling (1866–1927).

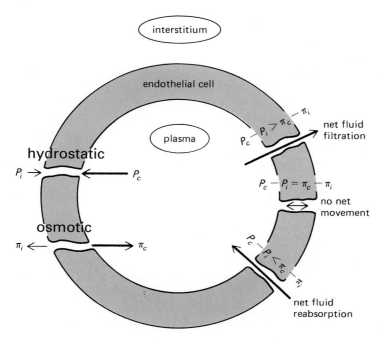

Figure 1-5   Factors influencing transcapillary fluid movement.

where P_c = the hydrostatic pressure of intracapillary fluid
$\quad\quad \pi_c$ = the oncotic pressure of intracapillary fluid
P_i and π_i = the same quantities for interstitial fluid
$\quad\quad K$ = a constant expressing how readily fluid can move across capillaries
(essentially the reciprocal of the resistance to fluid flow through the
capillary wall)

Fluid balance within a tissue (or the absence of net transcapillary water movement) occurs when the bracketed term in this equation is zero. This equilibrium may be upset by alterations in any of the four pressure terms. The pressure imbalances which cause capillary filtration and reabsorption are indicated on the right side of Fig. 1-5. In most tissues, rapid net filtration of fluid is abnormal. For example, a substance called histamine is often released in damaged tissue. One of the actions of histamine is to increase capillary permeability to the extent that protein leaks into the interstitium. Net filtration and tissue swelling (edema) accompany histamine release, in part because the oncotic pressure difference $(\pi_c - \pi_i)$ is reduced below normal.

Transcapillary fluid filtration is not necessarily detrimental. Indeed, fluid-producing organs such as salivary glands and kidneys utilize high intracapillary hydrostatic pressure to produce continual net filtration. Moreover, in certain abnormal situations, such as severe loss of blood volume through hemorrhage, the net fluid reabsorption accompanying diminished intracapillary hydrostatic pressure helps to restore the volume of circulating fluid.

A complicating fact is that intracapillary hydrostatic pressure is higher at the entrance to a capillary than it is at the exit because of pressure losses due to resistance as the blood flows along capillaries. At the beginning of capillaries the capillary hydrostatic pressure normally exceeds the capillary oncotic pressure, whereas the reverse is true near the venous end of capillaries. Thus there is normally net fluid filtration in the beginning portions of capillaries and net fluid reabsorption in the final portions. A whole capillary, then, is in "net" equilibrium when its initial filtration and later reabsorption are equal. Fortunately, the net transcapillary fluid movement can be evaluated by using the average value of intracapillary hydrostatic pressure in the Starling equation as we have shown in the preceding discussion.

LYMPHATIC SYSTEM

Despite the extremely low capillary permeability to proteins, these molecules as well as other large particles such as long-chain fatty acids and bacteria find their way into the interstitial space. If such particles were allowed to accumulate in the interstitial space, filtration forces would ultimately exceed reabsorption forces and edema would result. The lymphatic system represents a pathway by which large molecules reenter the circulating blood.

The lymphatic system begins in the tissues with blind-end lymphatic capillaries, which are roughly equivalent in size to but less numerous than regular capillaries. These capillaries are very porous and easily collect large particles accompanied by interstitial fluid. This fluid, called *lymph,* moves through the converging lymphatic vessels, is filtered through lymph nodes where bacteria and particulate matter are removed, and reenters the circulatory system near the point where the blood enters the right heart.

Flow of lymph from the tissues toward the entry point into the circulatory system is promoted by two factors: (1) increases in tissue interstitial pressure (due to fluid accumulation or to movement of surrounding tissue) and (2) contractions of the lymphatic vessels themselves. Valves located in these vessels also prevent backward flow.

Roughly 2.5 liters of lymphatic fluid enter the cardiovascular system each day. In the steady state, this indicates a total body *net* transcapillary fluid filtration rate of 2.5 liters per day. When compared to the total amount of blood that circulates each day (about 7000 liters), this may seem like an insignificant amount of net capillary fluid leakage. However, lymphatic blockage is a very serious problem and is accompanied by severe swelling. Thus the lymphatics play a critical role in keeping the interstitial protein concentration low and in removing excess capillary filtrate from the tissues.

Study Questions: 1 to 6

2

BASIC CARDIAC STRUCTURE AND FUNCTION

OBJECTIVES

The student understands the basic structure and function of the heart:

1 Identifies the chambers and valves of the heart and describes the pathway of blood flow through the heart.
2 Describes the pathway of action potential propagation in the heart.
3 Identifies the distribution of sympathetic and parasympathetic nerves in the heart and lists the basic effects of these nerves on the heart.
4 Lists five factors essential to proper ventricular pumping action.

PUMPING ACTION OF THE HEART

The heart lies in the center of the thoracic cavity suspended by its attachments to the great vessels within a thin fibrous sac called the *pericardium*. A small amount of fluid in the sac lubricates the surface of the heart and allows it to move freely during contraction and relaxation. The sole function of the heart is to supply the energy required for the circulation of blood in the cardiovascular system. Blood flow through all organs is passive and occurs only because arterial pressure is kept higher than venous pressure by the pumping action of the heart. The right heart pump provides the energy necessary to move blood through the pulmonary vessels and the left heart pump provides the energy that causes flow through the systemic organs.

The pathway of blood flow through the chambers of the heart is indicated in Fig. 2-1. Venous blood returns from the systemic organs to the right atrium via the superior and inferior venae cavae. It passes through the *tricuspid valve* into the right ventricle and from there is pumped through the *pulmonic valve* into the pulmonary circulation via the pulmonary arteries. Oxygenated pulmonary venous blood flows in pulmonary veins to the left atrium and passes through the *mitral valve* into the left ventricle. From there it is pumped through the *aortic valve* into the aorta to be distributed to the systemic organs.

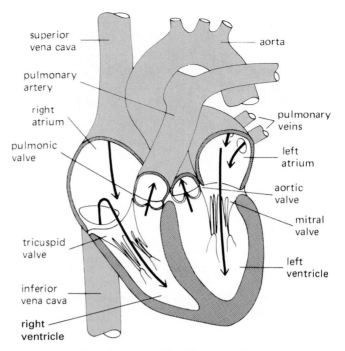

Figure 2-1   Pathway of blood flow through the heart.

Although the gross anatomy of the right heart pump is somewhat different from that of the left heart pump, the pumping principles are identical. Each pump consists of a ventricle which is a closed chamber surrounded by a muscular wall, as illustrated in Fig. 2-2. The valves are structurally designed to allow flow in only one direction and passively open and close in response to the direction of the pressure differences across them. Ventricular pumping action occurs because the volume of the intraventricular chamber is cyclically changed by rhythmic and synchronized contraction and relaxation of the individual cardiac muscle cells that lie in a circumferential orientation within the ventricular wall. When the ventricular muscle cells are contracting, they generate a circumferential tension in the ventricular walls which causes the pressure within the chamber to increase. As soon as the ventricular pressure exceeds the pressure in the pulmonary artery (right pump) or aorta (left pump), blood is forced out of the chamber through the outlet valve as shown in Fig. 2-2. This phase of the cardiac cycle during which the ventricular muscle cells are contracting is called *systole*. Because the pressure is higher in the ventricle than in the atrium during systole, the atrioventricular (AV) valve is closed. When the ventricular muscle cells relax, the pressure in the ventricle falls below that in the atrium, the AV valve opens, and the ventricle refills with blood as shown on the right of Fig. 2-2. This

VENTRICULAR SYSTOLE **VENTRICULAR DIASTOLE**

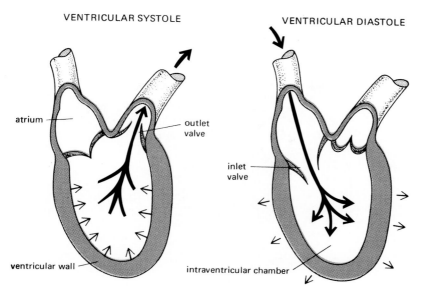

Figure 2-2 Ventricular pumping action.

portion of the cardiac cycle is called *diastole.* The outlet valve is closed during diastole because arterial pressure is greater than intraventricular pressure. After the period of diastolic filling, the systolic phase of a new cardiac cycle is initiated.

EXCITATION OF THE HEART

Efficient pumping action of the heart requires a precise coordination of the contraction of millions of individual cardiac muscle cells. Contraction of each cell is triggered when an electrical excitatory impulse (*action potential*) sweeps over its membrane. Proper coordination of the contractile activity of the individual cardiac muscle cells is achieved primarily by the conduction of this action potential from one cell to the next via gap junctions that connect all cells of the heart into a functional syncytium (i.e., acting as one synchronous unit). In addition, muscle cells in certain areas of the heart are specifically adapted to control the frequency of cardiac excitation, the pathway of conduction, and the rate of the impulse propagation through various regions of the heart. The major components of this specialized excitation and conduction system are shown in Fig. 2-3. They include the *sinoatrial node* (SA node), the atrial internodal tracts, the *atrioventricular node* (AV node), the common AV nodal *bundle of His,* and the right and left *bundle branches* made up of specialized cells called *Purkinje* fibers.

The SA node is located at the junction of the superior vena cava and the right atrium. The specialized atrial muscle cells of this region can spontaneously

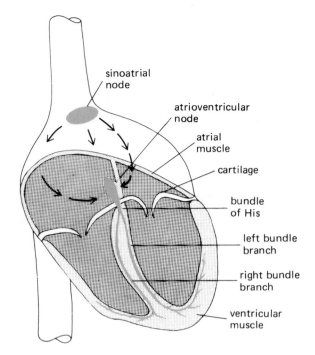

Figure 2-3   Electrical conduction system of the heart.

generate action potentials which are then propagated through the rest of the heart to cause cardiac contraction. This SA node region normally acts as the intrinsic cardiac pacemaker. The action potential then spreads through the atrial wall in a wave centered at the SA node. Although there is some evidence for preferred conduction pathways in the atria from the SA node to the AV node via anterior, middle, and posterior internodal bands, these pathways are not anatomically well-defined. The atrial conduction velocity is about 1 m/s, and the wave front of the action potential reaches the AV node roughly 0.08 s after having been generated in the SA node.

The AV node consists of small specialized cells located on the right side of the atrial septum just under the endocardium. The lower portion of the AV node consists of parallel fibers that normally form the only bridge of contiguous cardiac cells crossing the cartilaginous structure that provides support for the cardiac valves and electrically separates atria from ventricles. Propagation of the impulse through this AV nodal region is very slow (~0.05 m/s) and therefore a delay of ~0.15 s is imposed between excitation of the atria and the ventricles.

As the bundle of His enters the interventricular septum, it splits into a left bundle branch and a right bundle branch which are made up of large diameter Purkinje fibers. These specialized muscle fibers rapidly conduct the impulse at

~3 m/s down the septum to the subendocardial layers of the myocardium, the base of the papillary muscles, and, via penetrating fibers, to the epicardial regions of the right and left ventricular myocardium. The excitation wave traveling in the multiple branches of the Purkinje fibers ultimately is transferred to ordinary muscle cells. This results in rapid, very nearly simultaneous excitation of all ventricular muscle cells.

NEURAL INFLUENCES ON THE HEART

While the heart inherently beats on its own, cardiac function can be influenced profoundly by neural inputs from both the sympathetic and parasympathetic divisions of the autonomic nervous system. These inputs allow us to modify cardiac pumping as is appropriate to meet changing homeostatic needs of the body. All portions of the heart are richly innervated by *adrenergic sympathetic fibers.* When active, these sympathetic nerves release *norepinephrine* (noradrenaline) on cardiac cells. Norepinephrine interacts with beta adrenergic receptors on cardiac muscle cells to increase heart rate, increase action potential conduction velocity, and increase force of contraction. Overall, sympathetic activation acts to increase cardiac pumping.

Cholinergic parasympathetic nerve fibers travel to the heart via the vagus nerve and innervate the SA node, the AV node, and atrial muscle. When active, these parasympathetic nerves release *acetylcholine* on cardiac muscle cells. Acetylcholine interacts with *muscarinic* receptors on cardiac muscle cells to decrease heart rate (SA node) and decrease action potential conduction velocity (AV node). Parasympathetic nerves may also act to decrease the force of contraction of atrial (not ventricular) muscle cells. Overall, parasympathetic activation acts to decrease cardiac pumping. Usually an increase in parasympathetic nerve activity is accompanied by a decrease in sympathetic nerve activity, and vice-versa.

REQUIREMENTS FOR EFFECTIVE CARDIAC PUMPING

For effective efficient ventricular pumping action, the heart must be functioning properly in five basic respects:

1 The contractions of individual cardiac muscle cells must occur at regular intervals and be synchronized (not *arrhythmic*).
2 The valves must open fully (not *stenotic*).
3 The valves must not leak (not be *insufficient* or *regurgitant*).
4 The muscle contractions must be forceful (not *failing*).
5 The ventricles must fill adequately during diastole.

In the subsequent chapters, we shall study in detail how these requirements are met in the normal heart.

3

CHARACTERISTICS OF CARDIAC CELLS

OBJECTIVES

The student understands the ionic basis of the spontaneous electrical activity of cardiac muscle cells:

1 Describes how membrane potentials are created across semipermeable membranes by transmembrane ion concentration differences.
2 Defines equilibrium potential and knows its normal value for potassium and sodium ions.
3 States how membrane potential reflects a membrane's relative permeability to various ions.
4 Defines resting potential and action potential.
5 Describes the characteristics of "fast" and "slow" response action potentials.
6 Identifies the refractory periods of the cardiac cell electrical cycle.
7 Defines threshold potential and describes the interaction between ion channel conditions, and membrane potential during the depolarization phase of the action potential.
8 Defines pacemaker potential and describes the basis for rhythmic electrical activity of cardiac cells.
9 Lists the phases of the cardiac cell electrical cycle and states the membrane permeability alterations responsible for each phase.

The student knows the normal process of cardiac electrical excitation:

10 Describes gap junctions and their role in cardiac excitation.
11 Describes the normal pathway of action potential conduction through the heart.
12 Indicates the timing with which various areas of the heart are electrically excited and identifies the characteristic action potential shapes and conduction velocities in each major part of the conduction system.
13 States the relationship between electrical events of cardiac excitation and

the P, QRS, and T waves, the PR interval, and the ST segment of the electrocardiogram.

The student understands the factors that control heart rate and action potential conduction in the heart:

14 States how diastolic potentials of pacemaker cells can be altered to produce changes in heart rate.
15 Describes how cardiac sympathetic and parasympathetic nerves alter heart rate and conduction of cardiac action potentials.
16 Defines the terms *chronotropic* and *dromotropic*.

The student understands the contractile processes of cardiac muscle cells:

17 Describes the subcellular structures responsible for cardiac muscle cell contraction.
18 Defines and describes the excitation-contraction process.
19 Defines isometric, isotonic, and afterloaded contractions of cardiac muscle.
20 Describes the influence of altered preload on the tension-producing and shortening capabilities of cardiac muscle.
21 Describes the influence of altered afterload on the shortening capabilities of cardiac muscle.
22 Defines the terms *contractility* and *inotropic state* and describes the influence of altered contractility on the tension-producing and shortening capabilities of cardiac muscle.
23 Describes the effect of altered sympathetic neural activity on cardiac inotropic state.

ELECTRICAL ACTIVITY OF THE HEART

In all striated muscle cells, contraction is triggered by a rapid voltage change, called an *action potential*, that occurs on the cell membrane. Cardiac muscle cell action potentials differ sharply from those of skeletal muscle cells in three important ways that promote synchronous rhythmic excitation of the heart: (1) they can be self-generating; (2) they can be conducted directly from cell to cell; and (3) they have long durations, which preclude fusion of individual twitch contractions. To understand these special electrical properties of cardiac muscle and how cardiac function depends on them, we must first review the basic electrical properties of excitable cell membranes.

Membrane Potentials

All cells have an electrical potential (voltage) across their membranes. Such *membrane potentials* exist because the ionic concentrations of the cytoplasm are different from those of the interstitium and ions diffusing down concentration gradients across semipermeable membranes generate electrical gradients. For our purposes, the three most important ions to consider are sodium (Na^+) and calcium (Ca^{2+}) ions, which are more concentrated in the interstitial fluid than they are inside cells, and potassium (K^+) ions which have the opposite distribution. The diffusion of ions across the cell membrane occurs through *channels* that (1) are made up of protein molecules that span the membrane; (2) are specific for an individual ion (e.g., Na^+ channels), and (3) exist in various configurations that are either open, closed, or inactivated (unable to be opened). The *permeability* of the membrane to a specific ion is directly related to the number of channels for that ion that are open at a given instant in time.

Figure 3-1 shows how ion concentration differences can generate an electrical potential across the cell membrane. Consider first, as shown at the top of this figure, a cell that (1) has K^+ more concentrated inside the cell than out, (2) is permeable only to K^+ (i.e., only K^+ channels are open), and (3) has no initial transmembrane potential. Because of the concentration difference, K^+ ions (positive charges) will diffuse out of the cell. Meanwhile, negative charges, such as protein anions, cannot leave the cell because the membrane is impermeable to them. Thus the K^+ efflux will make the inside of the cell more electrically negative (deficient in positively charged ions) and at the same time make the interstitium more electrically positive (rich in positive ions). Now K^+, being positively charged, is attracted to regions of electrical negativity. Therefore when K^+ diffuses out of a cell, it creates an electrical potential across the membrane that tends to attract it back into the cell. There exists one membrane potential called the *potassium equilibrium potential* at which the electrical forces tending to pull K^+ into the cell exactly balance the concentration forces tending to drive K^+ out. When the membrane potential has this value, there is no net movement of K^+ across the membrane. With the normal concentrations of about 145 mM K^+ inside cells and 4 mM K^+ in the extracellular fluid, the K^+ equilibrium potential is roughly -90 mV (inside more negative than outside by nine-hundredths of a

ELECTRICAL ACTIVITY OF THE HEART

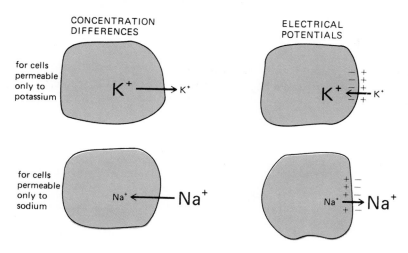

Figure 3-1   Electrochemical basis of membrane potentials.

volt).[1] A membrane that is permeable only to K^+ will inherently and rapidly (essentially instantaneously) develop the potassium equilibrium potential. In addition, membrane potential changes require the movement of so few ions that concentration differences are not significantly affected by the process.

As depicted in the bottom half of Fig. 3-1, similar reasoning shows how a membrane permeable only to Na^+ would have the *sodium equilibrium potential* across it. The sodium equilibrium potential is approximately +70 mV with the normal extracellular Na^+ concentration of 140 mM and intracellular concentration of 10 mM. Real cell membranes, however, are never permeable to just Na^+ or just K^+. When a membrane is permeable to both of these ions, the membrane potential will lie somewhere between the Na^+ equilibrium potential and the K^+ equilibrium potential. Just what membrane potential will exist any instant depends on the relative permeability of the membrane to Na^+ and K^+. The more permeable the membrane to K^+ than to Na^+, the closer the membrane potential will be to −90 mV. Conversely, when the permeability to Na^+ is high relative to the permeability to K^+, the membrane potential will be closer to +70 mV.[2] Because of low or unchanging permeabilities or low concentration, roles played by ions other than Na^+ and K^+ in determining membrane potential are usually minor and often ignored. However, as we shall see later, calcium ion, Ca^{2+}, do participate in the cardiac muscle action potential. Like Na^+, Ca^{2+} is more concentrated outside cells than inside. The equilibrium potential for Ca^{2+} is $\sim +100$ mV, and the cell membrane tends to become more positive on the inside when the membrane's permeability to Ca^{2+} rises.

Under resting conditions, most heart muscle cells have membrane potentials that are quite close to the potassium equilibrium potential. Thus both electrical and concentration gradients favor Na^+ entry into the resting cell. However, the very low permeability of the resting membrane to Na^+ in combination with an energy-requiring sodium pump that extrudes Na^+ from the cell prevents Na^+ from gradually accumulating inside the resting cell.[3]

---

[1] The equilibrium potential (E_{eq}) for any ion (X^z) is determined by its intracellular and extracellular concentrations as indicated in the Nernst equation:

$$E_{eq} = \frac{-61.5 \text{ mV}}{z} \log_{10} \frac{[X^z] \text{ inside}}{[X^z] \text{ outside}}$$

[2] A quantitative description of how Na^+ and K^+ concentrations and the relative permeability (P_{Na}/P_K) to these ions affect membrane potential (E_m) is given by the following equation:

$$E_m = -61.5 \text{ mV} \log_{10} \left(\frac{[K^+]_i + P_{Na}/P_K [Na^+]_i}{[K^+]_o + P_{Na}/P_K [Na^+]_o} \right)$$

[3] The sodium pump not only removes Na^+ from the cell but also pumps K^+ into the cell. Since more Na^+ is pumped out than K^+ is pumped in (3:2), the pump is said to be *electrogenic*. The resting membrane potential becomes slightly less negative than normal when the pump is abruptly inhibited.

Cardiac Cell Action Potentials

Action potentials of cells from different regions of the heart are not identical but have varying characteristics that are important to the overall process of cardiac excitation.

Some cells within the specialized conduction system have the ability to act as pacemakers and to spontaneously initiate action potentials whereas ordinary cardiac muscle cells do not (except under unusual conditions). Basic membrane electrical features of an ordinary cardiac muscle cell and a cardiac pacemaker-type cell are shown in Fig. 3-2. Action potentials from these cell types are referred to as

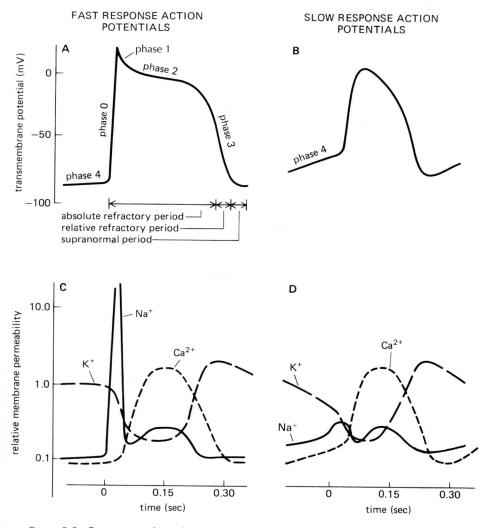

Figure 3-2   Time course of membrane potential and ion permeability changes that occur during "fast response" (left) and "slow response" (right) action potentials.

"fast response" or "slow response" action potentials, respectively. As shown in panel A of this figure, fast response action potentials are characterized by a rapid depolarization (phase 0) with a substantial overshoot (positive inside voltage), a rapid reversal of the overshoot potential (phase 1), a long plateau (phase 2), and a repolarization (phase 3) to a stable, high (i.e., large negative) resting membrane potential (phase 4). In comparison, the slow response action potentials, as shown in panel B, are characterized by a slower initial depolarization phase, a lower amplitude overshoot, a shorter and less stable plateau phase, and a repolarization to an unstable, slowly depolarizing "resting" potential. The unstable resting potential seen in pacemaker cells with slow response action potentials is variously referred to as the *phase 4 depolarization, diastolic depolarization,* or *pacemaker potential.*

As indicated at the bottom of Fig. 3-2A, cells are in an absolute refractory state during most of the action potential, i.e., they cannot be stimulated to fire another action potential. Near the end of the action potential, the membrane is relatively refractory and can be reexcited only by a larger than normal stimulus. Immediately after the action potential, the membrane is transiently hyperexcitable and is said to be in a "vulnerable" or "supranormal" period. Similar alterations in membrane excitability probably occur during slow action potentials but at present are not fully characterized.

Recall that the membrane potential of any cell at a particular instant in time depends on the relative permeability of the cell's membrane to specific ions at that instant. As in all excitable cells, cardiac cell action potentials are the result of transient changes in the ionic permeability of the cell membrane which are triggered by an initial depolarization. Panels C and D of Fig. 3-2 indicate the changes in membrane permeabilities to K^+, Na^+, and Ca^{2+}, which produce the various phases of the fast and slow response action potentials. Note that during the resting phase, the membranes of both types of cells are more permeable to K^+ than to Na^+ or Ca^{2+}. Therefore the membrane potentials are close to the potassium equilibrium potential (of -90 mV) during this period. In the pacemaker-type cells, at least three mechanisms are thought to contribute to the slow depolarization of the membrane observed during the diastolic interval. First, there is a progressive decrease in the membrane's permeability to K^+ during the resting phase, and second, the permeability to Na^+ increases slightly. The gradual increase in the Na^+/K^+ permeability ratio will cause the membrane potential to move slowly away from the K^+ equilibrium potential (-90 mV) in the direction of the Na^+ equilibrium potential. Third, there is an increase in the permeability of the membrane to calcium ions, which results in an inward movement of positively charged ions and also contributes to the diastolic depolarization.[4]

When the membrane potential depolarizes to a certain threshold potential in either type of cell, major rapid alterations in the permeability of the membrane to specific ions are triggered. Once initiated, these permeability changes cannot be stopped and they proceed to completion.

---

[4] Drugs acting as calcium channel blockers often result in a decrease in cardiac automaticity because of their inhibitory effects on this inward-going calcium current.

The characteristic rapid rising phase of the fast response action potential is a result of a sudden increase in Na^+ permeability. This produces what is referred to as the *fast inward current* of Na^+ and causes the membrane potential to move rapidly toward the sodium equilibrium potential. As indicated in panel *C* of Fig. 3-2, this period of very high sodium permeability is short-lived. It is followed by a more slowly developed increase in the membrane's permeability to Ca^{2+} and a decrease in its permeability to K^+. Also, there is a second slowly developing increase in Na^+ permeability which is thought to be caused by a different mechanism than that involved in the initial rapid Na^+ permeability changes. These more persistent permeability changes (which produce what is referred to as the *slow inward current*) prolong the depolarized state of the membrane to cause the plateau (phase 2) of the cardiac action potential. The initial fast inward current is small (or even absent) in cells that have slow response action potentials. The slow rising phase of these action potentials is therefore primarily a result of an inward movement of Ca^{2+} ions. In both types of cells, the membrane is repolarized (phase 3) to its original resting potential as the K^+ permeability increases and the Ca^{2+} and Na^+ permeabilities return to their low resting values. These late permeability changes produce what is referred to as the *delayed outward current*. .

The overall smoothly-graded permeability changes that produce action potentials are the net result of alterations in each of the many individual ion channels within the plasma membrane of a single cell. An experimental advancement called *patch clamping* has made it possible to study the operation of individual ion channels. The patch clamp data clearly indicate that a single channel is either open or closed at any instant in time; there are no graded states of partial opening. What is graded is the percentage of time that a channel spends in the open state, i.e., its probability of being open. While a channel may remain closed for long periods, it rarely remains open for more than a few milliseconds at a time. Thus, the probability of a channel's being open depends both on the *frequency* with which it opens and how long it remains open after each opening. An increase in an ion channel's probability of being open (channel "activation") leads to an increase in total open time and an increase in the overall membrane permeability to that ion.

Certain types of channels are called *voltage-gated channels* (or voltage-operated channels) because their probability of being open varies with membrane potential. Other types of channels, called *ligand-gated channels* (or receptor-operated channels), are activated by certain neurotransmitters or other specific signal molecules. Table 3-1 lists some of the major currents and channel types involved in cardiac cell electrical activity.

Some of the voltage-gated channels respond to a sudden onset, sustained change in membrane potential by only a brief period of activation. However, changes in membrane potential of slower onset but the same magnitude may fail to activate these channels at all. To explain such behavior, it is postulated that these channels have two independently operating "gates"—an *activation gate* and an *inactivation gate*—both of which must be open for the channel as a

Table 3-1   Characteristics of Important Cardiac Ion Channels in Order of Their
Participation in an Action Potential

Current	Channel	Gating mechanism	Functional role
i_{K1}	K+ channel (inward rectifier)	Voltage	Maintains high K+ permeability during phase 4 Its decay contributes to diastolic depolarization Its suppression during phases 0 to 2 contribute to plateau
i_{Na}	Na+ channel (fast)	Voltage	Accounts for phase 0 of action potential Inactivation may contribute to phase 1 of action potential
i_{to}	K+ channel (transient outward)	Voltage	Contributes to phase 1 of action potential
i_{Ca}	Ca2+ channel (slow, L channels)	Voltage	Primarily responsible for phase 2 of action potential Inactivation may contribute to phase 3 of action potential Is enhanced by sympathetic stimulation and β-adrenergic agents
i_K	K+ channel (delayed rectifier)	Voltage	Causes phase 3 of action potential May be enhanced by increased intracellular Ca2+
i_{KATP}	K+ channel (ATP-sensitive)	Ligand	Increases K+ permeability when [ATP] is low
i_{KACh}	K+ channel (acetylcholine-activated)	Ligand	Responsible for effects of vagal stimulation Decreases diastolic depolarization (and heart rate) Hyperpolarizes resting membrane potential Shortens phase 2 of the action potential
i_f ("funny")	Na+ channel (pacemaker current)	Both	Contributes to the diastolic depolarization Is enhanced by sympathetic stimulation and β-adrenergic agents Is suppressed by vagal stimulation

whole to be open. These gates both respond to changes in membrane potential but do so with different voltage sensitivities and time courses.

These concepts are illustrated in Fig. 3-3. In the resting state, with the membrane polarized to near -80 mV, the activation or m gate of the fast Na+ channel is closed, but its inactivation or h gate is open (Fig. 3-3A). With a rapid depolarization of the membrane to threshold, the Na+ channels will be activated strongly

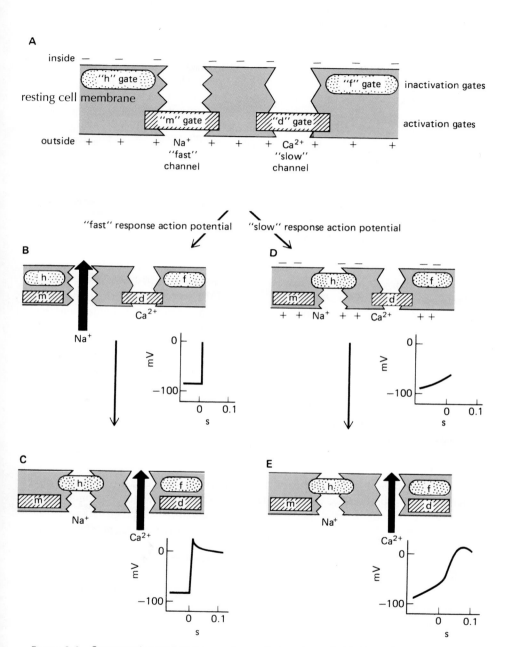

Figure 3-3 Conceptual model of changes in specific ion channels (A) during fast response (B and C) and slow response (D and E) action potentials.

to allow an inrush of positive sodium ions that further depolarizes the membrane and thus initiates a "fast" response action potential as illustrated in Fig. 3-3B. This occurs because the m gate responds to membrane depolarization by opening more quickly than the h gate responds by closing. Thus a rapid depolarization to threshold is followed by a brief but strong period of Na^+ channel activation wherein the m gate is open but the h gate has yet to close. In fact, phase 0 of the fast response cardiac action potential represents how rapidly the m gates can open, whereas phase 1 may, in part, represent the time course of h gate closure.

The initial membrane depolarization also causes the activation (d) gate of the Ca^{2+} channel to open after a brief delay. This permits the slow inward current of Ca^{2+} ions which help maintain the depolarization through the plateau phase of the action potential (Fig. 3-3C). Ultimately, repolarization occurs because of both a delayed inactivation of the Ca^{2+} channel (by closure of the f gates) and an opening of K^+ channels which are not shown in Fig. 3-3. The factors controlling the operation of the K^+ channels (which can be selectively blocked by tetraethylammonium ions) are not well understood. High intracellular Ca^{2+} concentration may be responsible for the activation of the K^+ channels during repolarization. The h gate remains closed during the remainder of the action potential, effectively inactivating the Na^+ channel and contributing to the long cardiac refractory period which lasts until the end of phase 3. With repolarization, both gates of the sodium channel return to their original position and the channel is now ready to be reactivated by a subsequent depolarization.

The slow response action potential shown in the right half of Fig. 3-3 differs from the fast response action potential primarily because of the lack of a strong activation of the fast Na^+ channel at its onset. This is a direct consequence of a slow depolarization to the threshold potential. Slow depolarization gives the inactivating h gates time to close even as the activating m gates are opening (Fig. 3-3D). Thus in a slow action potential, there is no initial period where all the sodium channels of a cell are essentially open at once. The depolarization beyond threshold is slow and caused primarily by the influx of Ca^{2+} through slow channels (Fig. 3-3E).

While cells in certain areas of the heart typically have fast-type action potentials and cells in other areas normally have slow-type action potentials, it is important to recognize that all cardiac cells are potentially capable of having either type of action potential depending on how fast they depolarize to the threshold potential. As we shall see, rapid depolarization to the threshold potential is usually an event forced on a cell by the occurrence of an action potential in an adjacent cell. Slow depolarization to threshold occurs when a cell itself spontaneously and gradually loses its resting polarization which normally happens only in the sinoatrial (SA) node. A *chronic* moderate depolarization of the resting membrane (caused, for example, by high extracellular K^+ concentration) can inactivate the fast channels (by closing the h gates) without inactivating the slow Ca^{2+} channels. Under these conditions, all cardiac cell action potentials will be of the slow type. Large sustained depolarizations, however, can inactivate both the fast and slow channels and thus make the cardiac muscle cells inexcitable.

Conduction of Cardiac Action Potentials

Action potentials are conducted over the surface of individual cells because active depolarization in any one area of the membrane produces local currents in the intracellular and extracellular fluids which passively depolarize immediately adjacent areas of the membrane to their voltage threshold for active depolarization.

Action potentials are propagated from cell to cell in the heart because adjacent heart muscle cells have regions of close membrane association called *gap junctions* (nexuses) through which the local internal electrical currents can easily pass. Specialized channels made of the protein connexin are present at the ends of the cells and join end to end to form an intercellular channel which allows ions to flow between cells. Figure 3-4 shows schematically how these gap junctions allow action potential propagation from cell to cell.

Cells B, C, and D are shown in the resting phase with more negative charges on the inside than the outside. Cell A is shown in the plateau phase of an action potential and has more positive charges inside than out. Because of the gap junctions, electrostatic attraction can cause a local current flow (ion movement) between the depolarized membrane of active cell A and the polarized membrane of resting cell B, as indicated by the arrows in the figure. This ion movement tends to eliminate the charge difference across the resting membrane; i.e., it depolarizes the membrane of cell B. Once the local currents from active cell A depolarize the membrane of cell B near the gap junction to the threshold level, an action potential will be triggered at that site and will be conducted over cell B. Because cell B branches (a common morphological characteristic of cardiac muscle fibers), its action potential will evoke action potentials on cells C and D. This process is continued through the entire myocardium.

The speed at which an action potential propagates through a region of cardiac tissue is called the *conduction velocity*. The conduction velocity varies considerably in different areas in the heart. This velocity is directly dependent on the diameter of the muscle fiber involved. Thus, conduction over small-diameter cells in the atrioventricular (AV) node is significantly slower than conduction

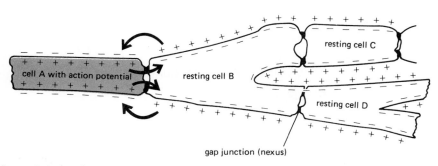

Figure 3-4   Local currents and cell-to-cell conduction of cardiac muscle cell action potentials.

over large-diameter cells in the ventricular Purkinje system. Conduction velocity is also directly dependent on the intensity of the local depolarizing currents which are in turn directly determined by the rate of rise of the action potential. Rapid depolarization favors rapid conduction. Variations in the capacitive and/or resistive properties of the cell membranes, gap junctions, and cytoplasm are also factors that contribute to the differences in conduction velocity of action potentials through specific areas of the heart.

Specific electrical adaptations of various cells in the heart are reflected in the characteristic shape of their action potentials, as shown in the right half of Fig. 3-5. Note that the action potentials shown in Fig. 3-5 have been positioned to indicate the time at which the electrical impulse that originates in the SA node reaches other areas of the heart. Cells of the SA node act as the heart's normal pacemaker and determine the heart rate. This is because the spontaneous depolarization of the resting membrane is most rapid in SA nodal cells, and they reach their threshold potential before cells elsewhere.

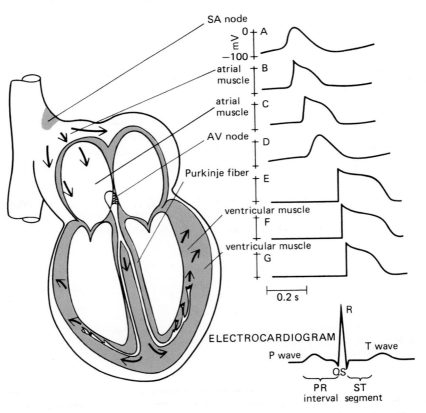

Figure 3-5 Electrical activity of the heart: single-cell voltage recordings (traces A to G) and lead II electrocardiogram.

The action potential initiated by an SA nodal cell first spreads progressively through the atrial wall. Action potentials from cells in two different regions of the atria are shown in Fig. 3-5: one close to the SA node and one more distant from the SA node. Both cells have similarly shaped action potentials, but their temporal displacement reflects the fact that it takes some time for the impulse to spread over the atria.

As shown in Fig. 3-5, cells of the AV node have action potentials similar in shape to those of SA nodal cells. Note also that AV nodal cells have a faster spontaneous resting depolarization than other cells of the heart except those in the SA node. The AV node is sometimes referred to as a *latent pacemaker*, and in many pathological situations it, rather than the SA node, controls the heart rhythm. Because of the small size of the nodal cells and the slow rate of rise of their action potentials, the cardiac impulse travels very slowly through the AV nodal tissue. Since the AV node delays the transfer of the cardiac impulse from the atria to the ventricles, the ventricles contract slightly after the atria in each cardiac cycle. Because of sharply rising action potentials and other factors, such as large cell diameters, electrical conduction is extremely rapid in Purkinje fibers. This allows the Purkinje system to transfer the cardiac impulse to cells in many areas of the ventricle nearly in unison. Action potentials from muscle cells in two areas of the ventricle are shown in Fig. 3-5. Because of the high conduction velocity in ventricular tissue, there is only a small discrepancy in their time of onset. Note in Fig. 3-5 that the ventricular cells which are the last to depolarize have shorter duration action potentials and thus are the first to re-polarize.

Electrocardiogram

Fields of electrical potential caused by the electrical activity of the heart extend through the body tissue and may be measured with electrodes placed on the body surface. *Scalar electrocardiography* provides a record of how the voltage between two points on the body surface changes with time as a result of the electrical events of the cardiac cycle. At any instant of the cardiac cycle the electrocardiogram indicates the net electrical field that is the summation of many weak electrical fields being produced by voltage changes occurring on in-dividual cardiac cells at that instant. When a large number of cells are simulta-neously depolarizing or repolarizing, large voltages are observed on the electro-cardiogram. Since the electrical impulse spreads through the heart tissue in a stereotyped manner, the temporal pattern of voltage change recorded between two points on the body surface is also stereotyped and will repeat itself with each heart cycle.

The lower trace of Fig. 3-5 represents a typical recording of the voltage changes normally measured between the right arm and the left leg as the heart goes through one cycle of electrical excitation; this record is called a lead II electrocardiogram and will be discussed in detail in Chap. 5. The major fea-tures of an electrocardiogram are the *P wave*, the *QRS complex*, and the *T wave*.

The P wave corresponds to atrial depolarization, the QRS complex to ventricular depolarization, and the T wave to ventricular repolarization.

Control of Heart Rate

Normal rhythmic contractions of the heart occur because of spontaneous electrical pacemaker activity of cells in the SA node. The interval between heartbeats (and thus the heart rate) is determined by how long it takes the membranes of these pacemaker cells to spontaneously depolarize to the threshold level. The heart beats at a spontaneous or *intrinsic rate* (≈ 100 beats per minute) in the absence of any outside influences. Outside influences *are* required, however, to increase or decrease the heart rate from its intrinsic level.

The two most important outside influences on heart rate come from the autonomic nervous system. Fibers from both the sympathetic and parasympathetic divisions of the autonomic system terminate on cells in the SA node and these fibers can modify the intrinsic heart rate. Activating the cardiac sympathetic nerves (increasing cardiac sympathetic *tone*) increases the heart rate. Increasing cardiac parasympathetic tone slows the heart. As shown in Fig. 3-6, the parasympathetic and sympathetic nerves both influence heart rate by altering the

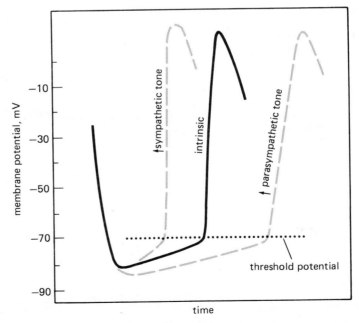

Figure 3-6   Effect of sympathetic and parasympathetic tone on pacemaker potential.

course of spontaneous depolarization of the resting potential in SA pacemaker cells.

Cardiac parasympathetic fibers, which travel to the heart through the *vagus* nerves, release the transmitter substance *acetylcholine* on SA nodal cells. Acetylcholine increases the permeability of the resting membrane to K^+ and decreases the diastolic permeability to Na^+.[5] As indicated in Fig. 3-6, these permeability changes have two effects on the resting potential of cardiac pacemaker cells: (1) they cause an initial hyperpolarization of the resting membrane potential by bringing it closer to the K^+ equilibrium potential and (2) they slow the rate of spontaneous depolarization of the resting membrane. Both these effects increase the time between beats by prolonging the time required for the resting membrane to depolarize to the threshold level. Since there is normally some continuous *tonic* activity of cardiac parasympathetic nerves, the normal resting heart rate is approximately 70 beats per minute.

Sympathetic nerves release the transmitter substance *norepinephrine* on cardiac cells. In addition to other effects discussed later, norepinephrine increases the inward currents carried by Na^+ (i_f) and by Ca^{2+} during the diastolic interval.[6] These changes will increase heart rate by increasing the rate of diastolic depolarization as shown in Fig. 3-6.

In addition to sympathetic and parasympathetic nerves, there are many (usually less important) factors that can alter heart rate. These include a number of ions and circulating hormones, as well as physical influences such as temperature and atrial wall stretch. All act by somehow altering the time required for the resting membrane to depolarize to the threshold potential. An abnormally high concentration of Ca^{2+} in the extracellular fluid, for example, tends to decrease heart rate by shifting the threshold potential. Factors that increase heart rate are said to have a *positive chronotropic effect*. Those that decrease heart rate have a *negative chronotropic effect*.

Besides their effect on heart rate, autonomic fibers also influence the conduction velocity of action potentials through the heart. Increases in sympathetic activity increase conduction velocity (have a *positive dromotropic effect*), whereas increases in parasympathetic activity decrease conduction velocity (have a *negative dromotropic effect*). These effects are most notable at the AV node and can influence the duration of the PR interval.

---

[5] The acetylcholine interacts with a muscarinic receptor on the SA nodal cell membrane which in turn is linked to an inhibitory G protein, G_i. The activation of G_i has two effects: (1) an increase in K^+ conductance resulting from an increased opening of the K_{ACh} channels and (2) a suppression of adenylate cyclase leading to a fall in intracellular cyclic adenosine monophosphate (cAMP) which reduces the inward-going pacemaker current carried by Na^+ (i_f).

[6] The norepinephrine interacts with a β_1-adrenergic receptor on the SA nodal cell membrane which in turn is linked to a stimulatory G protein, G_s. The activation of G_s increases adenylate cyclase, leading to an increase in intracellular cyclic AMP which increases the open-state probability of the pacemaker Na^+ current channel (i_f).

MECHANICAL ACTIVITY OF THE HEART

Cardiac Muscle Contraction

Contraction of the cardiac muscle cell is initiated by the action potential signal acting on intracellular organelles to evoke tension generation and/or shortening of the cell. In this section, we shall describe (1) the subcellular processes involved in coupling the excitation to the contraction of the cell (E-C coupling) and (2) the mechanical properties of cardiac cells.

Basic histological features of cardiac muscle cells are quite similar to those of skeletal muscle cells and include: (1) an extensive myofibrillar structure made up of parallel interdigitating thick and thin filaments arranged in serial units called *sarcomeres*, which are responsible for the mechanical processes of shortening and tension development[7]; (2) an internal compartmentation of the cytoplasm by an intracellular membrane system called the *sarcoplasmic reticulum* (SR), which sequesters calcium during the diastolic interval with the help of the calcium-storage protein, calsequestrin; (3) regularly spaced extensive invaginations of the cell membrane (sarcolemma), called *T tubules*, which appear to be connected to parts of the sarcoplasmic reticulum ("junctional" SR) by dense strands ("feet") and which carry the action potential signal to the inner parts of the cell; and (4) large numbers of mitochondria that provide the oxidative phosphorylation pathways needed to assure a ready supply of ATP to meet the high metabolic needs of cardiac muscle. The student is encouraged to consult a histology textbook for specific cellular morphological details.

Excitation-Contraction Coupling

Muscle action potentials trigger mechanical contraction through a process called *excitation-contraction coupling*, which is illustrated in Fig. 3-7. The major event of excitation-contraction coupling is a dramatic rise in the intracellular free Ca^{2+} concentration. The "resting" intracellular free Ca^{2+} concentration is less than 0.1 μM. In contrast, during maximum activation of the contractile apparatus, the intracellular free Ca^{2+} concentration reaches nearly 100 μM. When the wave of

---

[7] Proteins making up the thick and thin filaments are collectively referred to as "contractile proteins." The *thick filament* consists of a protein called *myosin*, which has a long straight tail with two globular heads each of which contains an adenosine triphosphate (ATP)-binding site and an actin-binding site; light chains are loosely associated with the heads and their phosphorylation may regulate (or modulate) muscle function. The *thin filament* consists of several proteins including *actin*—two α-helical strands of polymerized subunits (g-actin) with sites that interact with the heads of myosin molecules to form cross-bridges with the thick filaments; *tropomyosin*—a regulatory fibrous-type protein lying in the groove of the actin α helix which prevents actin from interacting with myosin when the muscle is at rest; and *troponin*—a regulatory protein consisting of three subunits: *troponin C*, which binds calcium ions during activation and initiates the configurational changes in the regulatory proteins that expose the actin site for cross-bridge formation; *troponin T*, which anchors the troponin complex to tropomyosin; and *troponin I*, which participates in the inhibition of actin-myosin interaction at rest.

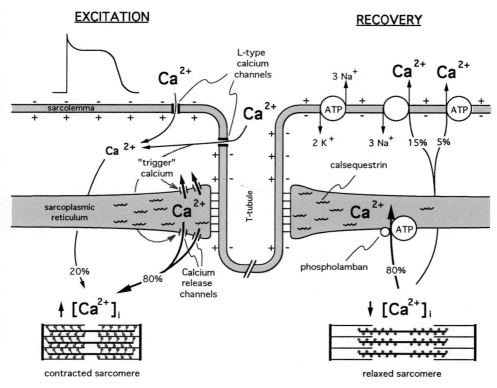

Figure 3-7   Excitation-contraction coupling and sarcomere shortening.

depolarization passes over the muscle cell membrane and down the T tubules, Ca^{2+} is released from the sarcoplasmic reticulum into the intracellular fluid.

As indicated on the left side of Fig. 3-7, the specific trigger for this release appears to be the entry of calcium into the cell via the L-type calcium channels and an increase in Ca^{2+} concentration in the region just under the sarcolemma on the surface of the cell and throughout the t-tubular system. Unlike skeletal muscle, this highly localized increase in calcium is essential for triggering the massive release of calcium from the SR. This *calcium-induced calcium release* is a result of opening calcium-sensitive release channels on the SR.[8] Although the amount of Ca^{2+} that enters the cell during a single action potential is quite small compared to that released from the SR, it is not only essential for triggering the SR calcium release but also essential for maintaining adequate levels of Ca^{2+} in the intracellular stores over the long run.

When the intracellular Ca^{2+} level is high ($>1.0\mu M$), links called *cross-*

---

[8]   These channels may be blocked by the plant alkaloid, ryanodine, and are activated by the methylxanthine, caffeine. These agents are chemical tools used to assess properties of these SR channels.

bridges form between two types of filaments found within muscle. Sarcomere units, as depicted in the lower part of Fig. 3-7, are joined end to end at Z lines to form *myofibrils*, which run the length of the muscle cell. During contraction, thick and thin filaments slide past one another to shorten each sarcomere and thus the muscle as a whole. The bridges form when the regularly spaced myosin heads from thick filaments attach to regularly spaced sites on the actin molecules in the thin filaments. Subsequent deformation of the bridges result in a pulling of the actin molecules toward the center of the sarcomere. This actin-myosin interaction requires energy from adenosine triphosphate (ATP). In resting muscles, the attachment of myosin to the actin sites is inhibited by troponin and tropomyosin. Calcium causes muscle contraction by interacting with troponin C to cause a configurational change that removes the inhibition of the actin sites on the thin filament. Since a single cross-bridge is a very short structure, gross muscle shortening requires that cross-bridges repetitively form, produce incremental movement between the myofilaments, detach, form again at a new actin site, and so on, in a cyclic manner.

There are several processes that participate in the reduction of intracellular Ca^{2+} that terminates the contraction. These processes are illustrated on the right side of Fig. 3-7. Approximately 80 percent of the calcium is actively taken back up into the SR by the action of Ca^{2+}-ATPase pumps located in the network part of the SR.[9] About 20 percent of the calcium is extruded from the cell into the extracellular fluid either via the Na^+-Ca^{2+} exchanger located in the sarcolemma[10] or via sarcolemmal Ca^{2+}-ATPase pumps.

Excitation-contraction coupling in cardiac muscle is different from that in skeletal muscle in that it may be modulated; different intensities of actin-myosin interaction (contraction) can result from a single action potential trigger in cardiac muscle. The mechanism for this seems to be dependent upon variations in the amount of Ca^{2+} reaching the myofilaments and therefore the number of cross-bridges activated during the twitch. This ability of cardiac muscle to vary its contractile strength—i.e., change its *contractility*—is extremely important to cardiac function, as will be discussed in a later section of this chapter.

The duration of the cardiac muscle cell contraction is approximately the same as that of its action potential. Therefore, the electrical refractory period of a cardiac muscle cell is not over until the mechanical response is completed. As

---

[9]   The action of these pumps is regulated by the protein, phospholamban. When this protein is phosphorylated the rate of Ca^{2+} resequestration is increased and the rate of relaxation is enhanced.

[10] The Na^+-Ca^{2+} exchanger is powered by the sodium gradient across the sarcolemma which in turn is maintained by the Na^+/K^+ ATPase. This exchanger is electrogenic in that three Na^+ ions move into the cell in exchange for each Ca^{2+} ion that moves out. This net inward movement of positive charge may contribute to the maintenance of the plateau phase of the action potential. The cardiac glycoside, digitalis, slows down the Na^+/K^+ pump and thus reduces the sodium gradient which in turn results in an increase in intracellular Ca^{2+}. This mechanism contributes to the positive effect of cardiac glycosides on the contractile force of the failing heart.

a consequence, heart muscle cells cannot be activated rapidly enough to cause a fused (tetanic) state of prolonged contraction. This is fortunate because intermittent contraction and relaxation are essential for the heart's pumping action.

Cardiac Muscle Cell Mechanics

The cross-bridge interaction which occurs after a muscle is activated to contract gives the muscle the potential to develop force and/or shorten. Whether it does one, the other, or some combination of the two depends primarily on what is allowed to happen by the external constraints placed on the muscle during the contraction. For example, activating a muscle whose ends are held rigidly causes it to develop tension, but it cannot shorten. This is called an *isometric* ("fixed length") contraction. The force that a muscle produces during an isometric contraction indicates its maximum ability to develop tension. At the other extreme, activating an unrestrained muscle causes it to shorten without force development because it has nothing to develop force against. This type of contraction is called an *isotonic* ("fixed tension") contraction. Under such conditions, a muscle shortens with its maximum possible velocity (called V_{max}), which is determined by the maximum possible rate of cross-bridge cycling. Adding load to the muscle decreases the velocity and extent of its shortening. Thus, the course of a muscle contraction depends both on the inherent capabilities of the muscle and the external constraints placed on the muscle during contraction. Muscle cells in the ventricular wall operate under different constraints during different phases of each cardiac cycle. To understand ventricular function, we must first examine how cardiac muscle behaves when constrained in several different ways.

Isometric Contractions: Length-Tension Relationships The influence of muscle length on the behavior of cardiac muscle during isometric contraction is illustrated in Fig. 3-8. The top panel shows the experimental arrangement for measuring muscle force at rest and during contraction at three different lengths. The middle panel shows time records of muscle tensions recorded at each of the three lengths, and the bottom panel shows a graph of the tension results plotted against muscle length.

The first important fact illustrated in Fig. 3-8 is that force is required to stretch a resting muscle to different lengths. This force is called the *resting tension*. The lower curve in the graph in Fig. 3-8 shows the resting tension measured at different muscle lengths and is referred to as the *resting length-tension curve*. When a muscle is stimulated to contract while its length is held constant, it develops an additional component of tension called *active tension*. The *total tension* exerted by a muscle during contraction is the sum of the active and resting tensions.

The second important fact illustrated in Fig. 3-8 is that the active tension developed by cardiac muscle during the course of an isometric contraction de-

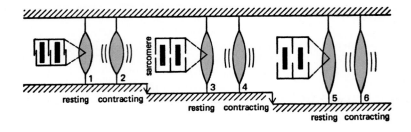

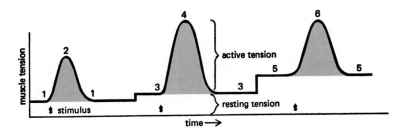

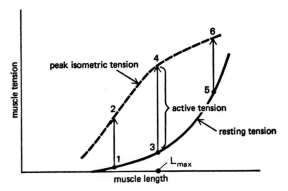

Figure 3-8   Isometric contractions and the effect of muscle length on resting tension and active tension development.

pends very much on the muscle length at which the contraction occurs. Active tension development is maximum at some intermediate length referred to as L_{max}. Little active tension is developed at very short or very long muscle lengths. Normally, cardiac muscle operates at lengths well below L_{max}, so that increasing muscle length increases the tension developed during an isometric contraction.

There are three separate mechanisms that have been proposed to explain the relationship between muscle length and developed tension. The first mechanism to be identified suggests that this relationship depends on the *extent of overlap* of the thick and thin filaments in the sarcomere at rest. Histological studies indicate that the changes in the resting length of the whole muscle are associated with proportional changes in the individual sarcomeres. Peak tension development occurs at sarcomere lengths of 2.2 to 2.3 μm. At sarcomere lengths shorter than ~ 2.0 μm, the opposing thin filaments may overlap or buckle and thus interfere with active tension development as shown at the top of Fig. 3-8. At long sarcomere lengths, overlap may be insufficient for optimal cross-bridge formation.

The second (and perhaps most important) mechanism is based on a length-dependent change in *sensitivity* of the myofilaments to calcium. At short lengths only a fraction of the potential cross-bridges are apparently activated by a given increase in intracellular calcium. At longer lengths, more of the cross-bridges become activated leading to an increase in active tension development. This change in calcium sensivitity occurs immediately after a change in length with no time delay. The "sensor" responsible for the length-dependent activation of cardiac muscle seems to reside with the troponin C molecule, but how it happens is not fully understood.

The third mechanism rests on the observation that within several minutes after increasing the resting length of cardiac muscle, there is an increase in the *amount* of calcium that is released with excitation, which is coupled to a further increase in force development. It is thought that stretch-sensitive ion channels in the cell membranes may be responsible for this delayed response.

To what extent each of these mechanisms is contributing to the contractile force of the cardiac muscle at any instant is not clear, nor very important for our purposes. In any case, the dependence of active tension development on muscle length is a fundamental property of cardiac muscle that has extremely important effects of heart function.

Isotonic and Aferloaded Contractions   During what is termed *isotonic* ("fixed load") contraction, a muscle shortens against a constant load. A muscle contracts isotonically when lifting a fixed weight such as the 1-g load shown in Fig. 3-9. Such a 1-g weight placed on a resting muscle will result in some specific resting muscle length, which is determined by the muscle's resting length-tension curve. If the muscle were to contract isometrically at this length, it would be capable of generating a certain amount of tension, e.g., 4.5 g as indicated by the dashed line in the graph of Fig. 3-9. A contractile tension of 4.5 g obviously cannot be generated while lifting a 1-g weight. When a muscle has contractile potential in excess of the tension it is actually developing, it shortens. Thus in an isotonic contraction, muscle length decreases at constant tension, as illustrated by the horizontal arrow from point 1 to point 3 in Fig. 3-9. As the muscle shortens, however, its contractile potential inherently decreases, as indicated by the downward slope of the peak isometric tension curve in Fig. 3-9. There exists some short length at which the muscle is capable of generating only 1 g of tension, and when this length is reached, shortening must

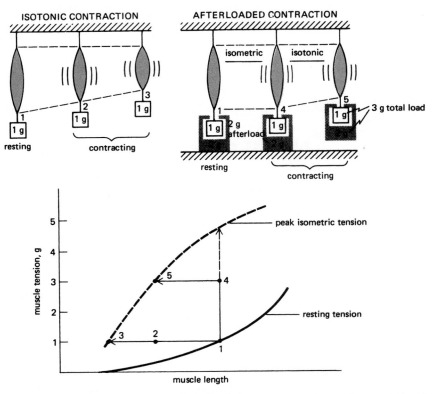

Figure 3-9   Relationship of isotonic and afterloaded contractions to the cardiac muscle length-tension diagram.

cease.[11] Thus the curve on the cardiac muscle length-tension diagram that indicates how much isometric tension a muscle can develop at various lengths also establishes the limit on how far muscle shortening can proceed with different loads.

Figure 3-9 also shows a complex type of muscle contraction called an *afterloaded isotonic contraction*, in which the load on the muscle at rest, the *preload*, and the load on the muscle during contraction, the *total load*, are different. In the example of Fig. 3-9 the preload is equal to 1 g, and because an additional 2-g weight (the *afterload*) is engaged during contraction, the total load equals 3 g.

---

[11] In reality, muscle shortening requires some time and the duration of a muscle twitch contraction is limited because intracellular Ca^{2+} levels are elevated only briefly following the initiation of a membrane action potential. For this and possibly other reasons, isotonic shortening may not actually proceed quite as far as the isometric tension development curve on the length-tension diagram suggests is possible. Since this complication does not alter the general correspondence between a muscle's isometric and isotonic performance, we choose to ignore it.

Since preload determines the resting muscle length, both isotonic contractions shown in Fig. 3-9 begin from the same length. Because of the different loading arrangement, however, the afterloaded muscle must increase its total tension to 3 g before it can shorten. This initial tension will be developed isometrically and can be represented as going from point 1 to point 4 on the length-tension diagram. Once the muscle generates enough tension to equal the total load, its tension output is fixed at 3 g and it will now shorten isotonically because its contractile potential still exceeds its tension output. This isotonic shortening is represented as a horizontal movement on the length-tension diagram along the line from point 4 to point 5. As in any isotonic contraction, shortening must cease when the muscle's tension-producing potential is decreased sufficiently by the length change to be equal to the load on the muscle. Note that the afterloaded muscle shortens less than the nonafterloaded muscle even though both muscles began contracting at the same initial length. The factors that affect the extent of cardiac muscle shortening during an afterloaded contraction are of special interest to us, because, as we shall see, stroke volume is determined by how far cardiac muscle shortens under these conditions.

Cardiac Muscle Contractility   A number of factors in addition to initial muscle length can affect the tension-generating potential of cardiac muscle. *Any intervention that increases the peak isometric tension that a muscle can develop at a* fixed length *is said to increase cardiac muscle contractility.* Such an agent is said to have a *positive inotropic effect* on the heart.

The most important physiological regulator of cardiac muscle contractility is norepinephrine. When norepinephrine is released on cardiac muscle cells from sympathetic nerves, it has not only the chronotropic effect on heart rate discussed earlier but also a pronounced positive inotropic effect that causes cardiac muscle cells to contract more rapidly and forcefully.

The positive effect of norepinephrine on the isometric tension-generating potential is illustrated in Fig. 3-10A. When norepinephrine is present in the solution bathing cardiac muscle, the muscle will, *at every length*, develop more isometric tension when stimulated than it would in the absence of norepinephrine. In short, norepinephrine raises the peak isometric tension curve on the cardiac muscle length-tension graph. Norepinephrine is said to increase cardiac muscle contractility because it enhances the forcefulness of muscle contraction *even when length is constant*. Changes in contractility and initial length can occur simultaneously, but by definition a change in *contracility* must involve a shift from one peak isometric length-tension curve to another.

Figure 3-10B shows how raising the peak isometric length-tension curve with norepinephrine increases the amount of shortening in afterloaded contractions of cardiac muscle. With preload and total load constant, more shortening occurs in the presence of norepinephrine that in its absence. This is because when contractility is increased, the tension-generating potential is equal to the total load at a shorter muscle length. Note that norepinephrine has no effect on the resting length-tension relationship of cardiac muscle. Thus norepinephrine

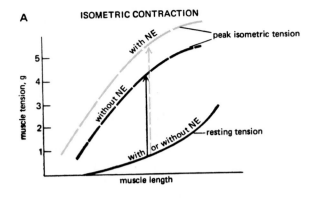

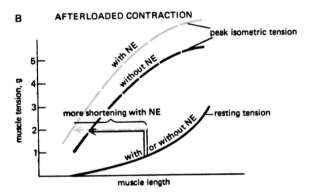

Figure 3-10   Effect of norepinephrine (NE) on isometric (A) and afterloaded (B) contractions of cardiac muscle.

causes increased shortening by changing the final but not the initial muscle length associated with afterloaded contractions.

The cellular mechanism of the norepinephrine effect on contractility is mediated by its interaction with a β_1-adrenergic receptor. The signalling pathway involves an activation of the G_s protein-cAMP-protein kinase A, which then phosphorylates the Ca^{2+} channel increasing the inward calcium current during the plateau of the action potential. This increase in calcium influx not only contributes to the magnitude of the rise in intracellular Ca^{2+} for a given beat but also loads the internal calcium stores, which allows more to be released during subsequent depolarizations. This increase in free Ca^{2+} during activation allows more cross-bridges to be formed and greater tension to be developed.

Since norepinephrine also causes phosphorylation of the regulatory protein, phospholamban, on the sarcoplasmic reticular Ca^{2+} ATPase pump, the rate of calcium retrapping into the SR is enhanced and the rate of relaxation is increased. This is called a *positive lusitropic effect*. Thus in the presence of cate-

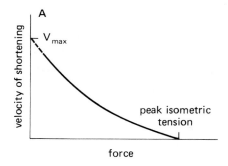

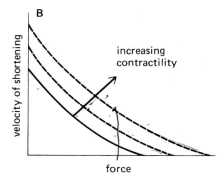

Figure 3-11   Cardiac muscle force-velocity relationship.

cholamines, systolic contraction is not only more forceful but also shorter in duration.[12,13]

Enhanced parasympathetic activity has been shown to have a small negative inotropic effect upon the heart. In the atria, where this effect is most pronounced, the negative inotropic effect is thought to be due to a shortening of the action potential and a decrease in the amount of Ca^{2+} that enters the cell during the action potential.

Changes in heart rate also influence cardiac contractility. Recall that a small amount of extracellular Ca^{2+} enters the cell during the plateau phase of each action potential. As the heart rate increases, more Ca^{2+} enters the cells per minute. There is a buildup of intracellular Ca^{2+} and a greater amount of Ca^{2+} is released into the sarcoplasm with each action potential. Thus, a sudden increase in beating rate is followed by a progressive increase in contractile force to a higher

[12]   Most catecholamine effects on the heart are a result of increases in sympathetic stimulation. Circulating catecholamines of adrenal origin are normally so low that their effects are negligible.

[13]   All of the effects of catecholamines on cardiac muscle can be blocked by specific drugs called *β-adrenergic receptor blocking agents*. These β-blockers are commonly used in the treatment of coronary artery disease to thwart the increased metabolic demands placed on the heart by the activity of sympathetic nerves.

plateau. This behavior is called the *staircase phenomenon* (or treppe). Changes in contractility produced by this intrinsic mechanism are sometimes referred to as *homeometric autoregulation*. The importance of such rate-dependent modulation of contractility in normal ventricular function is not clear at present.

The contractility of isolated cardiac muscle is often assessed by first determining the peak velocity of shortening of the preparation during isotonic contractions against several different total loads. The date obtained are used to construct what is known as the muscle *force-velocity* relationship as shown in Fig. 3-11A. The force-velocity relationship indicates the trade-off between force development and shortening velocity which is inherent in the contractile machinery of all muscle. The isometric force generating capability of the muscle is indicated by the point where the curve intersects the force axis. The point where the force-velocity curve intersects the velocity axis is called V_{max}. This V_{max} point has been shown to be closely correlated with the actin-myosin ATPase activity of the muscle and is thought to indicate the maximum possible rate of interaction between thick and thin filaments within the sarcomere. The V_{max} value is commonly used as an index of the contractility of isolated cardiac muscle. Fig. 3-11B shows the effect of norepinephrine (or other inotropic agents) on the force-velocity relationship. Note that both peak isometric tension and V_{max} increase with increases in the contracility of the preparation.

Study questions: 7 to 10

4

THE HEART PUMP

OBJECTIVES

The student knows the basic electrical and mechanical events of the cardiac cycle:

1 Correlates the electrocardiographic events with the mechanical events during the cardiac cycle.
2 Lists the major distinct phases of the cardiac cycle as delineated by valve opening and closure.
3 Describes the pressure and volume changes in the atria, the ventricles, and the aorta during each phase of the cardiac cycle.
4 Defines and states normal values for (1) ventricular end-diastolic volume, end-systolic volume, stroke volume, diastolic pressure, and peak systolic pressure, and (2) aortic diastolic pressure, systolic pressure, and pulse pressure.
5 States similarities and differences between mechanical events in the left and right heart pump.
6 States the origin of the heart sounds.

The student understands the factors that determine cardiac output:

7 States the relationship between cardiac output, heart rate, and stroke volume.
8 Identifies the major influences on heart rate.
9 Identifies the major determinants of stroke volume.
   a. Describes the relationship between ventricular wall tension, chamber radius, and pressure (the law of Laplace).
   b. Diagrams the relationship between left ventricular pressure and volume during the cardiac cycle.
   c. States the Frank-Starling law of the heart.
   d. Predicts the effect of altered ventricular preload on stroke volume and the ventricular pressure/volume relationship.
   e. Predicts the effect of altered ventricular afterload on stroke volume and the ventricular pressure/volume relationship.

f. Predicts the effect of altered ventricular contractility (inotropic state) on stroke volume and the ventricular pressure/volume relationship.

10 Summarizes the influences of the autonomic nervous system and alterations in cardiac pre- and afterload on cardiac output.

11 Describes the effect of cardiac sympathetic nerves on contractility, stroke volume, and cardiac output.

12 Draws a family of cardiac function curves describing the relationship between filling pressure and cardiac output under various levels of sympathetic tone.

13 Given data, calculates cardiac output using the Fick principle.

14 Identifies various imaging methods currently used to obtain clinical information about cardiac function.

The repetitive, synchronized contraction and relaxation of the cardiac muscle cells provides the forces necessary to pump blood through the systemic and pulmonary circulation. In this chapter, we shall describe (1) basic mechanical features of this cardiac pump, (2) factors that influence and/or regulate the cardiac output, and (3) various methods for estimating cardiac mechanical function.

CARDIAC CYCLE

Left Pump

The mechanical function of the heart can be described by the pressure, volume, and flow changes that occur within it during one cardiac cycle. A cardiac cycle is defined as one complete sequence of contraction and relaxation. The normal mechanical events of a cycle of the left heart pump are correlated in Fig. 4-1. This important figure summarizes a great deal of information and should be studied carefully.

Ventricular Diastole   The *diastolic phase*[1] of the cardiac cycle begins with the opening of the atrioventricular (AV) valves. As shown in Fig. 4-1, the mitral valve opens when left ventricular pressure falls below left atrial pressure and the period of ventricle filling begins. Blood that had previously accumulated in the atrium behind the closed mitral valve empties rapidly into the ventricle and this causes an initial drop in atrial pressure. Later, the pressures in both chambers slowly rise together as the atrium and ventricle continue filling in unison with blood returning to the heart through the veins.

Atrial contraction is initiated near the end of ventricular diastole by the depolarization of the atrial muscle cells, which causes the P wave of the electrocardiogram. As the atrial muscle cells develop tension and shorten, atrial pressure rises and an additional amount of blood is forced into the ventricle. At normal heart rates, atrial contraction is not essential for adequate ventricular filling. This is evident in Fig. 4-1 from the fact that the ventricle has nearly reached its maximum or *end-diastolic volume* before atrial contraction begins. Atrial contraction plays an increasingly significant role in ventricular filling as heart rate increases

---

[1]   The atria and ventricles do not beat simultaneously. Usually, and unless otherwise noted, systole and diastole denote phases of ventricular operation.

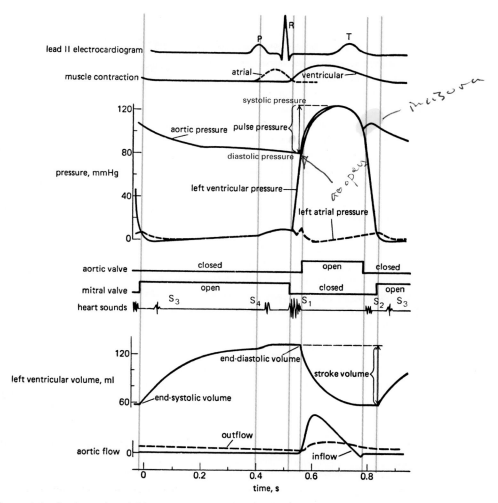

Figure 4-1 Cardiac cycle—left heart.

because the time interval between beats for passive filling becomes progressively shorter with increased heart rate. Note that throughout diastole, atrial and ventricular pressures are nearly identical. This is because a normal open mitral valve has very little resistance to flow and thus only a very small atrial-ventricular pressure difference is necessary to produce ventricular filling.

Ventricular Systole Ventricular systole begins when the action potential breaks through the AV node and sweeps over the ventricular muscle—an event heralded by the QRS complex of the electrocardiogram. Contraction of the ventricular muscle cells causes intraventricular pressure to rise above that in the atrium, which causes abrupt closure of the AV valve.

Pressure in the left ventricle continues to rise sharply as the ventricular contraction intensifies. When the left ventricular pressure exceeds that in the aorta, the aortic valve opens. The period of time between mitral valve closure and aortic valve opening is referred to as the *isovolumetric contraction phase* because during this interval the ventricle is a closed chamber with a fixed volume. Ventricular ejection begins with the opening of the aortic valve. In early ejection, blood enters the aorta rapidly and causes the pressure there to rise. Pressure builds simultaneously in both the ventricle and the aorta as the ventricular muscle cells continue to contract in early systole. This period is often called the *rapid ejection phase.*

Left ventricular and aortic pressure ultimately reach a maximum called *peak systolic pressure.* At this point the strength of ventricular muscle contraction begins to wane. Muscle shortening and ejection continue, but at a reduced rate. Aortic pressure begins to fall because blood is leaving the aorta and large arteries faster than blood is entering from the left ventricle. Throughout ejection, very small pressure differences exist between the left ventricle and the aorta because the aortic valve orifice is so large that it presents very little resistance to flow.

Eventually, the strength of the ventricular contraction diminishes to the point where intraventricular pressure falls below aortic pressure. This causes abrupt closure of the aortic valve. A dip, called the *incisura* or *dicrotic notch,* appears in the aortic pressure trace because a small volume of aortic blood must flow backward to fill the aortic valve leaflets as they close. Note that throughout ventricular systole, blood continues to return to the heart and fill the atrium. Thus atrial pressure progressively rises during ventricular systole to the high value that promotes rapid ventricular filling once the AV valve opens to begin the next heart cycle.

After aortic valve closure, intraventricular pressure falls rapidly as the ventricular muscle relaxes. For a brief interval, called the *isovolumetric relaxation period,* the mitral valve is also closed. Ultimately, intraventricular pressure falls below atrial pressure, the AV valve opens, and a new cardiac cycle begins. The ventricle has reached its minimum or *end-systolic volume* at the time of aortic valve closure. The amount of blood ejected from the ventricle during a single beat, the *stroke volume,* is equal to ventricular end-diastolic volume minus ventricular end-systolic volume.

The aorta distends or balloons out during systole because more blood enters the aorta than leaves it. During diastole, the arterial pressure is maintained by the elastic recoil of walls of the aorta and other large arteries. Nonetheless, aortic pressure gradually falls during diastole as the aorta supplies blood to the systemic vascular beds. The lowest aortic pressure, reached at the end of diastole, is called *diastolic pressure.* The difference between diastolic and peak systolic pressure in the aorta is called the arterial *pulse pressure.* Typical values for systolic and diastolic pressures in the aorta are 120 and 80 mmHg, respectively.

At a normal resting heart rate of about 70 beats per minute, the heart spends approximately two-thirds of the cardiac cycle in diastole and one-third in systole. When increases in heart rate occur, both diastolic and systolic intervals become shorter. Action potential durations are shortened and conduction velocity is increased. Contraction and relaxation rates are also enhanced. This shortening of the systolic interval tends to blunt the potential adverse effects of increases in heart rate on diastolic filling time.

Right Pump

Because the entire heart is served by a single electrical excitation system, similar mechanical events occur essentially simultaneously in both the left heart and the right heart. Both ventricles have synchronous systolic and diastolic periods and the valves of the right and left heart normally open and close nearly in unison. Since the two sides of the heart are arranged in series in the circulation, they must pump the same amount of blood and therefore must have identical stroke volumes.

The major difference between the right and left pumps is in the magnitude of the peak systolic pressure. The pressures developed by the right heart as shown in Fig. 4-2 are considerably lower than those for the left heart (Fig. 4-1). The lungs provide considerably less resistance to blood flow than that offered collectively by the systemic organs. Therefore less arterial pressure is required to drive the cardiac output through the lungs than is required through the systemic organs. Typical pulmonary artery systolic and diastolic pressures are 24 and 8 mmHg, respectively.

The pulsations that occur in the right atrium are transmitted in retrograde fashion to the large veins near the heart. These pulsations, shown on the atrial pressure trace of Fig. 4-2, can provide clinically useful information about the heart. Atrial contraction produces the first pressure peak called the *a* wave. The *c*

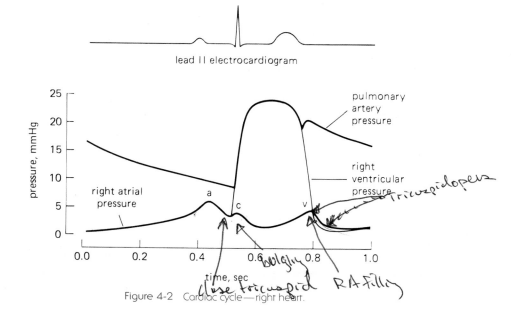

Figure 4-2 Cardiac cycle—right heart.

wave, which follows shortly thereafter, coincides with the onset of ventricular systole and is caused by an initial bulging of the tricuspid valve into the right atrium. Right atrial pressure falls after the c wave because of atrial relaxation and a downward displacement of the tricuspid valve during ventricular emptying. Right atrial pressure then begins to increase toward a third peak, the v wave, as the central veins and right atrium fill behind a closed tricuspid valve with blood returning to the heart from the peripheral organs. With the opening of the tricuspid valve at the conclusion of ventricular systole, right atrial pressure again falls as blood moves into the relaxed right ventricle. Shortly afterward, right atrial pressure begins to rise once more toward the next a wave as returning blood fills the central veins, the right atrium, and right ventricle together during diastole.

Heart Sounds

A phonocardiographic record of the heart sounds, which occur in the cardiac cycle, is included in Fig. 4-1. The first heart sound, S_1, occurs at the beginning of systole because of the abrupt closure of the AV valves, which produces vibrations of the cardiac structures and the blood in the ventricular chambers. S_1 can be heard most clearly by placing the stethoscope over the apex of the heart. Note that this sound occurs immediately after the QRS complex of the electrocardiogram.

The second heart sound, S_2, arises from the closure of the aortic and pulmonic valves at the beginning of the period of isovolumetric relaxation. This sound is heard at about the time of the T wave in the electrocardiogram. The pulmonic valve usually closes slightly after the aortic valve. Since this discrepancy is enhanced during the inspiratory phase of the respiratory cycle, inspiration causes what is referred to as the *physiological splitting of the second heard sound.* The discrepancy in valve closure during inspiration may range from 30 to 60 ms. One of the factors that leads to prolonged ejection of the right ventricle during inspiration is that the decreased intrathoracic pressure that accompanies inspiration transiently enhances venous return and diastolic filling of the right heart. For reasons that will be detailed later in this chapter, this extra filling volume will be ejected but a little extra time is required to do so. The aortic and pulmonic components of the second heart sound can best be heard by placing the stethoscope over the second intercostal space to the left and right of the sternum, respectively.

The third and fourth heart sounds are normally not detectable through a stethoscope. When they are present, however, they, along with S_1 and S_2, produce what are called *gallop rhythms* (resembling the sound of a galloping horse). When present, the third heart sound occurs shortly after S_2 during the period of rapid passive ventricular filling. Although S_3 may sometimes be detected in normal children, it is heard more commonly in patients with left ventricular failure *(ventricular gallop rhythm).* The fourth heart sound, which occasionally is heard shortly before S_1, is associated with atrial contraction and rapid active filling of the ventricle. Thus the combination of S_1, S_2, and S_4 sounds produces what is called an *atrial gallop rhythm*. The presence of S_4 often indicates an increased ventricular diastolic stiffness which can occur with several cardiac disease states.

CARDIAC OUTPUT

Cardiac output (liters of blood pumped by *each* of the ventricles per minute) is an extremely important cardiovascular variable that is continuously adjusted so that the cardiovascular system operates to meet the body's moment-to-moment transport needs. In going from rest to strenuous exercise, for example, the cardiac output of an average person will increase from approximately 5.8 to perhaps 15 liters/min. The extra cardiac output provides the exercising skeletal muscles with the additional nutritional supply needed to sustain an increased metabolic rate. To understand the cardiovascular system's response not only to exercise but to all other physiological or pathological demands placed on it, we must understand what determines and controls cardiac output.

Cardiac output (CO) is determined by the amount of blood ejected from each ventricle with each beat (the stroke volume, SV) and the number of heartbeats per minute (the heart rate, HR) as follows:

$$CO = HR \times SV$$
$$\frac{Volume}{Minute} = \frac{beats}{minute} \times \frac{volume}{beat}$$

It should be evident from this relationship that all influences on cardiac output must act by changing either heart rate or stroke volume.

Factors influencing heart rate do so by altering the characteristics of the diastolic depolarization of the pacemaker cells as discussed in Chap. 3 (Fig. 3-6). Recall that variations in activity of the sympathetic and parasympathetic nerves leading to cells of the SA node constitute the most important regulators of heart rate. Increases in sympathetic activity increase heart rate whereas increases in parasympathetic activity decrease heart rate. These neural inputs have immediate effects (within one beat) and therefore can cause very rapid adjustments in cardiac output.

CONTROL OF STROKE VOLUME
The Law of Laplace

Certain geometric factors dictate how the length-tension behavior of cardiac muscle fibers in the ventricular wall determines the volume-pressure behavior of the ventricular chamber. The actual relationships are complex because the shape of the ventricle is complex. The left ventricle is often modeled as either a cylinder or a sphere, although its actual shape lies somewhere in between the two. Since cardiac muscle cells are oriented circumferentially in the ventricular wall, either model can be used to illustrate three important functional points:

1   An increase in ventricular volume causes an increase in ventricular circumference and therefore an increase in the length of individual cardiac muscle cells (and vice-versa).
2   At any given ventricular volume, an increase in intraventricular pressure causes an increase in the tension on individual cardiac muscle cells in the wall (and vice-versa).
3   As ventricular volume increases (i.e., as the ventricular radius increases), a larger force is required from each individual muscle cell to produce any given intraventricular pressure.

The last point is a reflection of the *law of Laplace,* which is a statement of the relationship that exists between forces within the walls of any curved fluid container and pressure of its contents. If the ventricle is modeled as a cylinder where changes in ventricular volume occur only by changes in radius, the law of Laplace states that the total ventricular wall tension (T) per unit length of wall along the cylinder axis depends both on the intraventricular pressure (P) and intraventricular radius (r) as $T = P \cdot r$. This equation also applies to individual cardiac muscle cell tension because, in a cylindrical ventricular model, the number of muscle cells in a unit length is constant. (The law of Laplace takes on somewhat different forms for different vessel shapes but in all cases the implication is similar: wall tension is a function of both internal pressure and vessel radius.[2])

Figure 4-3 helps to illustrate how changes in muscle length and tension and ventricular pressure and volume that occur during the cardiac cycle are interrelated through the law of Laplace. Assume that diagram *A* in this figure indicates the state of the ventricle at the beginning of diastole. Its pressure, radius, and wall tension are related by $T = P \cdot r$. During diastole, ventricular radius (volume) increases with little increase in pressure. As indicated in the transition from *A* to *B* of the figure, doubling the radius at constant pressure would cause a doubling of wall tension because of the law of Laplace. During isovolumetric contraction, cardiac muscle fibers develop tension without shortening. As indicated by the transition from *B* to *C* in Fig. 4-3, a further 25-fold increase in wall tension at a constant radius will cause a 25-fold increase in intraventricular pressure because of the law of Laplace. During the initial phase of cardiac ejection, ventricular radius decreases while wall tension remains constant. The transition from *C* to *D* in Fig. 4-3 illustrates how a decrease in radius at constant wall tension is accompanied by a further increase in intraventricular pressure. Finally, the transition

---

[2]   With a spherical model, the law of Laplace states that $T = P \cdot r/2$ where again T is the total tension *per unit length* of wall. In the spherical ventricular model, however, a change in radius also changes the number of muscle cells contained in a unit length of the wall. When this is taken into account, the tension on each cell (T_{cell}) is related to ventricular pressure and radius as: $T_{cell} \propto P \cdot r^2$.

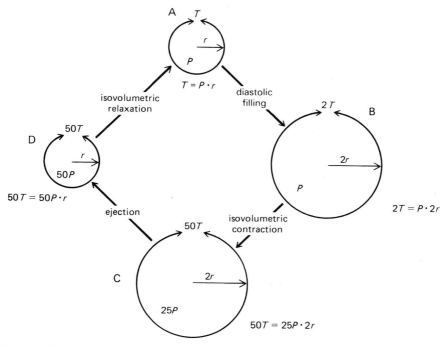

Figure 4-3 The law of Laplace and ventricular function in a cylindrical model. $P =$ intraventricular pressure; $r =$ intraventricular radius; $T =$ total wall tension in a unit length of the cylinder.

from D to A in Fig. 4-3 shows why pressure falls in the ventricle as a consequence of decreasing wall tension during isovolumetric relaxation.

A more complete description of the relationship between intraventricular pressure and volume changes which occur during a typical cardiac cycle is indicated in Fig. 4-4A, and the corresponding muscle length and tension changes are shown in Fig. 4-4B. (Figure 4-4A is simply another way of representing the intraventricular pressure and volume changes previously illustrated in Fig. 4-1. It is suggested that the student compare Fig. 4-4A with Fig. 4-1 until their interrelationship is clear.)

It is apparent from Fig. 4-4 that each major phase of the ventricular cardiac cycle has a corresponding phase of cardiac muscle length and tension change. During diastolic ventricular filling, for example, the progressive increases in ventricular pressure and volume combine to increase muscle tension $(T = P \cdot r)$, which passively stretches the resting cardiac muscle to greater lengths along its resting length-tension curve. End-diastolic pressure is referred to as *ventricular preload* because it sets the resting tension of the cardiac muscle fibers at the end of diastole.

At the onset of systole, the ventricular muscle cells develop tension isometrically and intraventricular pressure rises accordingly $(P = T/r)$. After the intraven-

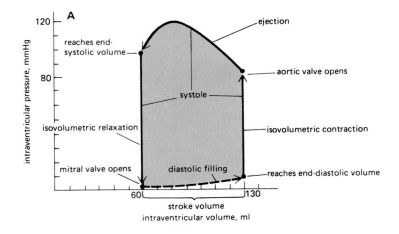

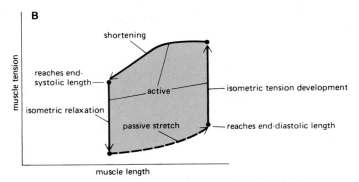

Figure 4-4   Ventricular pressure-volume cycle (A) and corresponding cardiac muscle length-tension cycle (B).

tricular pressure rises sufficiently to open the outlet valve, ventricular ejection begins as a consequence of ventricular muscle shortening. Systemic arterial pressure is often referred to as the *ventricular afterload* because it determines the tension that must be developed by cardiac muscle fibers before they can shorten.[3]

During cardiac ejection, cardiac muscle is simultaneously generating active tension and shortening. The magnitude of ventricular volume change during ejection (or stroke volume) is determined simply by how far ventricular muscle cells shorten during contraction. This, as we have already discussed, depends on

---

[3]   This designation is somewhat misleading for at least two reasons. First, arterial pressure is more analogous to ventricular total load than to ventricular afterload. Second, because of the law of Laplace, the actual wall tension that needs to be generated to attain a given intraventricular pressure also depends on the ventricular radius.

the length-tension relationship of the cardiac muscle cells and the load against which they are shortening. Once shortening ceases and the output valve closes, the cardiac muscle cells relax isometrically. Ventricular wall tension and intra-ventricular pressure fall in parallel during isovolumetric relaxation because the ventricular radius is constant throughout this final phase of systole.

Effect of Changes in Ventricular Preload: Frank-Starling Law of the Heart

The volume of blood that the heart ejects with each beat can vary significantly. One of the most fundamental causes of variations in stroke volume was described by William Howell in 1884 and by Otto Frank in 1894 and was formally stated by E. H. Starling in 1918. These investigators demonstrated that *the heart contracts more forcefully during systole when it is filled to a greater degree during diastole.* As a consequence, and as illustrated in Fig. 4-5, with other factors equal, *stroke volume increases as cardiac filling increases.* This phenomenon is referred to as the *Frank-Starling law of the heart.* We now recognize that the mechanical properties of myocardial muscle cells are the basis for the Frank-Starling law. Figure 4-6A illustrates how increasing muscle preload will increase the extent of shortening during a subsequent contraction with a fixed total load. Recall from the nature of the resting length-tension relationship that an increased preload is necessarily accompanied by increased initial muscle fiber length. When a muscle starts from a greater length, it has more room to shorten before it reaches the length at which its tension-generating capability equals the total load against which it must shorten. The same relationship exists for the muscle fiber when it is in place in the ventricle wall and results in the change in the ventricular pressure-volume loop shown in Fig. 4-6B. Increases in ventricular preload produce significant increases in stroke volume because longer initial fiber lengths greatly enhance the amount of muscle fiber

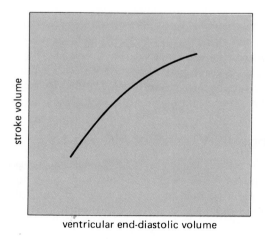

Figure 4-5   Frank-Starling law of the heart.

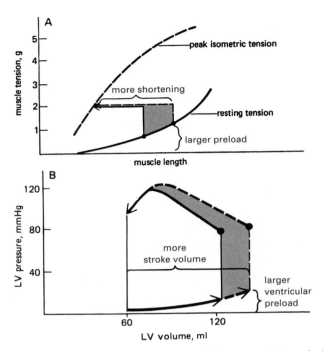

Figure 4-6 Effect of changes in preload on cardiac muscle shortening during afterloaded contractions (*A*) and on ventricular stroke volume (*B*).

shortening in an afterloaded contraction. This is the basis for the Frank-Starling law of the heart. Such preload-dependent regulation of stroke volume is sometimes referred to as *heterometric autoregulation.*

It should be noted in Fig. 4-6*A* that increasing preload increases initial muscle length without significantly changing the final length to which the muscle shortens against a constant total load. Thus increasing ventricular filling pressure increases stroke volume primarily by increasing end-diastolic volume. As shown in Fig. 4-6*B*, this is not accompanied by a significant increase in end-systolic volume because the enhanced strength of contraction that comes from larger end-diastolic volume through the Frank-Starling law ensures that the extra blood that enters the ventricle during diastole is ejected during systole.

Effect of Changes in Ventricular Afterload

Figure 4-7*A* shows how increased total load, at constant preload, has a negative effect on cardiac muscle shortening. Again, this is simply a consequence of the fact that muscle cannot shorten beyond the length at which its peak isometric tension-generating potential equals the total load upon it. Thus shortening must stop at a greater muscle length when total load is increased.

Normally, mean ventricular afterload is quite constant, because mean arte-

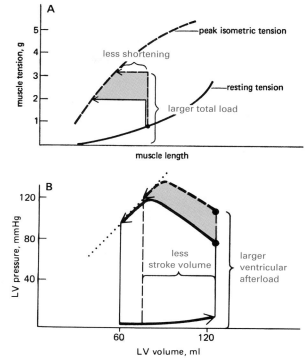

Figure 4-7   Effect of changes in afterload on cardiac muscle shortening during afterloaded contractions (A) and on ventricular stroke volume (B).

rial pressure is held within tight limits by the cardiovascular control mechanisms described later. In many pathological situations such as hypertension and aortic valve obstruction, however, ventricular function is adversely influenced by abnormally high ventricular afterload. When this occurs, stroke volume is decreased as shown by the changes in the pressure-volume loop in Fig. 4-7B. This change results from the decreased ability of the cardiac muscle cells to shorten against the increased afterload. Under these conditions, note that end-systolic volume is increased.

The relationship between end-systolic pressure and end-systolic volume obtained at a constant preload but different afterloads is indicated by the dotted line in Fig. 4-7B. This line can be thought of as roughly the ventricular pressure-volume equivalent of the muscle length-peak isometric tension curve. The slope of this line is being used clinically as an index of myocardial function as will be discussed in a later section of this chapter.

Effect of Changes in Cardiac Muscle Contractility

Recall that activation of the sympathetic nervous system results in release of norepinephrine from cardiac sympathetic nerves which increases contractility of the individual cardiac muscle cells. This results in an upward shift of the peak

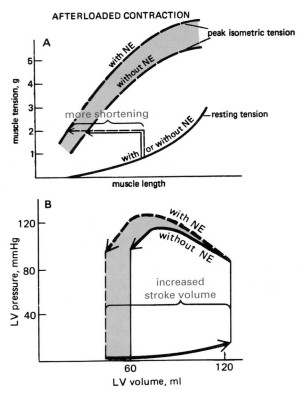

Figure 4-8 Effect of norepinephrine (NE) on afterloaded contractions on cardiac muscle (A) and on ventricular stroke volume (B).

isometric length-tension curve. As shown in Fig. 4-8A, such a shift will result in an increase in the shortening of a muscle contracting with constant preload and total load. Thus, as shown in Fig. 4-8B, the norepinephrine released by sympathetic nerve stimulation will increase ventricular stroke volume by decreasing the end-systolic volume without directly influencing the end-diastolic volume.

As previously discussed, the V_{max} value is commonly used as an index of the state of contractility of isolated cardiac muscle. Myocardial contractility cannot be directly measured in patients. However, several indirect methods are used to obtain clinically useful information about this important determinant of cardiac function. In one method, cardiac catheters are placed in the ventricle and the maximum rate of pressure development (dP/dt_{max}) during the isovolumetric contraction is measured. This is used as an index of contractility on the grounds that, in isolated cardiac muscle preparations, changes in contractility and V_{max} cause changes in the rate of tension development in an isometric contraction. Decreases in left ventricular dP/dt_{max} below the normal values of 1500 to 2000 mmHg/s indicate that myocardial contractility is below normal. Other methods of assessing contractility which use information derived from cardiac imaging techniques are discussed at the end of this chapter.

SUMMARY OF DETERMINANTS OF CARDIAC OUTPUT

The major influences on cardiac output that have been discussed in this chapter are summarized in Fig. 4-9. Heart rate is controlled by chronotropic influences on the spontaneous electrical activity of SA nodal cells. Cardiac parasympathetic nerves have a negative chronotropic effect, and sympathetic nerves have a positive chronotropic effect on the SA node. Stroke volume is controlled by influences on the contractile performance of ventricular cardiac muscle—in particular its degree of shortening in the afterloaded situation. The three distinct influences on stroke volume are contractility, preload, and afterload. Increased cardiac sympathetic nerve activity tends to increase stroke volume by increasing the contractility of cardiac muscle. Increased arterial pressure tends to decrease stroke volume by increasing the afterload on cardiac muscle fibers. Increased ventricular filling pressure increases end-diastolic volume, which tends to increase stroke volume through the Frank-Starling law.

It is important to recognize at this point that both heart rate and stroke volume are subject to more than one influence. Thus the fact that increased contractility tends to increase stroke volume should not be taken to mean that, in the intact cardiovascular system, stroke volume is always high when contractility is high. Following blood loss caused by hemorrhage, for example, stroke volume may be low in spite of a high level of sympathetic nerve activity. Still, the information presented in this chapter is directly applicable to all cardiovascular situations including hemorrhage. We can correctly reason, for example, that a high level of cardiac sympathetic nerve activity cannot be the cause of the low stroke volume accompa-

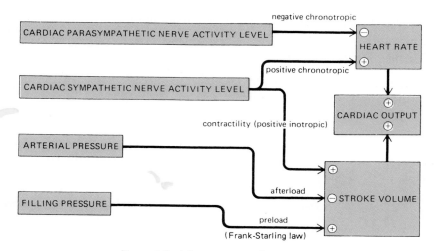

Figure 4-9   Influences on cardiac output.

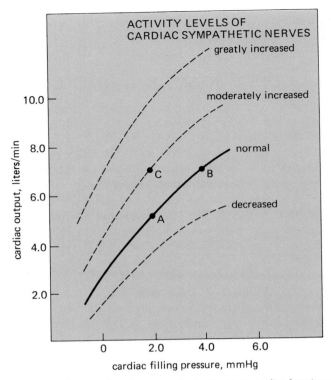

Figure 4-10   Influence of cardiac sympathetic nerves on cardiac function curves.

nying hemorrhage. The only other possible causes for low stroke volume are high arterial pressure or low cardiac filling pressure. Since arterial pressure is normal or low following hemorrhage, the low stroke volume associated with severe blood loss must be (and is) the result of low cardiac filling pressure.

Cardiac Function Curves

One very useful way to summarize the influences on cardiac function and the interactions between them is by *cardiac function curves* such as those shown in Fig. 4-10. In this case, cardiac output is treated as the dependent variable and is plotted on the vertical axis in Fig. 4-10, while cardiac filling pressure is plotted on the horizontal axis.[4] Different curves are used to show the influence of alterations in sympathetic nerve activity. Thus, Fig. 4-10 shows how the cardiac filling pressure and the activity level of cardiac sympathetic nerves interact to

---

[4]   Other variables may appear on the axes of these curves. The vertical axis may be designated as stroke volume or stroke work whereas the horizontal axis may be designated as central venous pressure, right (or left) atrial pressure, or ventricular end-diastolic volume (or pressure). In all cases, the curves describe the relationship between preload and cardiac function.

determine cardiac output. When cardiac filling pressure is 2 mmHg and the activity of cardiac sympathetic nerves is normal, the heart will operate at point A and will have a cardiac output of 5 liters/min. Each single curve in Fig. 4-10 shows how cardiac output would be changed by changes in cardiac filling pressure if cardiac sympathetic nerve activity were held at a fixed level. For example, if cardiac sympathetic nerve activity remained normal, increasing cardiac filling pressure from 2 to 4 mmHg would cause the heart to shift its operation from point A to point B on the cardiac function diagram. In this case, cardiac output would increase from 5 to 7 liters/min solely as a result of the increased filling pressure (the Frank-Starling law). If, on the other hand, cardiac filling pressure were fixed at 2 mmHg while the activity of cardiac sympathetic nerves was moderately increased from normal, the heart would change from operating at point A to operating at point C. Cardiac output would again increase from 5 to 7 liters/min. In this instance, however, cardiac output does not increase through the length-dependent mechanism because cardiac filling pressure did not change. Cardiac output increases at constant filling pressure with an increase in cardiac sympathetic activity for two reasons. First, increased cardiac sympathetic nerve activity increases heart rate. Second, but just as important, increased sympathetic nerve activity increases stroke volume by increasing cardiac contractility. Cardiac function graphs thus consolidate our knowledge of many mechanisms of cardiac control, and we will find them most helpful in understanding how the heart interacts with other elements in the cardiovascular system.

CARDIAC ENERGETICS
Energy Sources

In order for the heart to operate properly, it must have an adequate supply of chemical energy in the form of adenosine triphosphate (ATP). The substrates from which ATP can be formed by the heart may vary depending on which are in the greatest supply at a particular instant. For example, after a high carbohydrate meal, the heart will take up and metabolize glucose and pyruvate, whereas between meals, the heart can switch to metabolize free fatty acids, triglycerides, and ketones. Furthermore, glycogen is stored in myocardial cells as a reserve energy supply and can be mobilized via the glycolytic pathway to provide extra substrate under conditions of increased sympathetic stimulation. [Catecholamines interacting with membrane β receptors increase intracellular cyclic adenosine monophosphate (cAMP), which then activates phosphorylase b to stimulate glycogen metabolism.] The end-product of metabolism of glycogen, glucose, fatty acids, triglycerides, pyruvate, and lactate is acetyl CoA which enters the citric acid (Krebs) cycle in the mitochondria where, by a process of oxidative phosphorylation, the molecules are degraded to CO_2 and water and the energy is converted to ATP. (The student is encouraged to consult a biochemistry textbook for further details of these important metabolic pathways.)

The anaerobic sources of energy in the heart (e.g., glycolysis, creatine phosphate) are not adequate to sustain the metabolic demand for more than a few minutes. The heavy (nearly total) reliance of the heart on the aerobic pathways for ATP production is evident by (1) the high number of mitochondria in the cardiac muscle cells and (2) by the presence of high concentrations of the oxygen-binding protein, myoglobin, within the cardiac cells. Myoglobin can release its oxygen to the mitochondrial cytochrome oxidase system when intracellular oxygen levels are lowered. In these regards, cardiac muscle resembles "red" skeletal muscle that is adapted for sustained contractile activity as opposed to "white" skeletal muscle that is adapted for high-intensity, short-duration contractile activity.

Determinants of Myocardial Oxygen Consumption

In many pathological situations, such as obstructive coronary artery disease, the oxygen requirements of the myocardial tissue may exceed the capacity of coronary blood flow to deliver oxygen to the heart muscle. It is important, therefore, to understand what factors determine the myocardial oxygen consumption rate because reduction of the oxygen demand may be of significant clinical benefit to the patient.

Because the heart derives its energy almost entirely from aerobic metabolism, myocardial oxygen consumption is directly related to myocardial energy use (i.e., ATP splitting). Understanding the determinants of myocardial oxygen consumption essentially means understanding the myocardial processes that require ATP.

The *basal metabolism* of the heart tissue normally accounts for about 25 percent of myocardial ATP use and therefore myocardial oxygen consumption in a resting individual. Since basal metabolism represents the energy consumed in cellular processes other than contraction (e.g., energy-dependent ion pumping), little can be done to reduce it.

The processes associated with *muscle contraction* account for about 75 percent of myocardial energy use. Primarily this reflects ATP splitting associated with cross-bridge cycling during the isovolumetric contraction and ejection phases of the cardiac cycle. Some ATP is also used for CA^{2+} sequestration at the termination of each contraction.

The energy expended during the isovolumetric contraction phase of the cardiac cycle accounts for the largest portion (~ 50 percent) of total myocardial oxygen consumption despite the fact that the heart does no external work during this period. The energy needed for isovolumetric contraction depends heavily on the intraventricular pressure which must develop during this time, i.e., on the cardiac afterload. *Cardiac afterload* then is a major determinant of myocardial oxygen consumption. Reductions in cardiac afterload can produce clinically significant reductions in myocardial energy requirements and therefore myocardial oxygen consumption. Actually, energy utilization during isovolumetric contraction is more directly related to isometric *wall tension* development than to intraventricular pressure development. Recall that wall tension is related to intraventricular pressure *and* ventricular radius through the law of Laplace ($T = P \cdot r$). Consequently, reductions in cardiac preload (i.e., end-diastolic volume, radius) will also tend to reduce the energy required for isovolumetric contraction.

It is during the ejection phase of the cardiac cycle that the heart actually performs external work and the energy the heart expends during ejection depends on how much *external work* it is doing. In a fluid system, work (force × distance) is equal to pressure (force/distance^2) × volume (distance^3).[5] The external physical work done by the left ventricle in one beat, called *stroke work,* is equal to the area enclosed by the left ventricular pressure-volume loop (see Fig. 4-4). Stroke work is increased either by an increase in stroke volume (increased "volume" work) or by an increase in afterload (increased "pressure" work). In terms of ATP utilization and oxygen consumption, increases in the pressure work of the heart are more costly than increases in volume work. Thus, reductions in afterload are especially helpful in reducing the myocardial oxygen requirements for doing external work.

Changes in *myocardial contractility* can have important consequences on the oxygen requirement for basal metabolism, isovolumic wall tension generation, and external work. Heart muscle cells use more energy in rapidly developing a given tension and shortening by a given amount than in doing the same thing more slowly. Also, with increased contractility, more energy is expended in active Ca^{2+} transport. The net result of these influences is often referred to as the "energy wasting" effect of increased contractility.

Heart rate is also one of the more important determinants of myocardial oxygen consumption because the energy costs per minute must equal the energy cost per beat times the number of beats per minute. In general, it has been found that it is more efficient (less oxygen is required) to achieve a given cardiac output with low heart rate and high stroke volume than with high heart rate and low stroke volume. This again appears to be related to the relatively high energy cost of the pressure development phase of the cardiac cycle. The less pressure (wall tension) developed and the less often pressure development occurs, the better.

Many attempts have been made to develop clinically practical methods for estimating myocardial oxygen requirements from routinely measured cardiovascular variables. While none of these take into account all the factors that can influence myocardial oxygen consumption and therefore do not give 100 percent accurate predictions in all situations, many have proven to be of some usefulness. Perhaps the simplest "index" of the energy demands of the heart is obtained by multiplying peak systolic arterial pressure times heart rate. This *pressure-rate product* takes into account two of the most important factors in cardiac energy use (the magnitude and frequency of pressure development) and requires no invasive measures. Another formula, the *tension-time index,* is defined as summed areas under the systolic portions of a ventricular pressure recording for one minute. A continuous high-fidelity recording of intraventricular pressure such as that obtained during cardiac catheterization is required to calculate the tension-time

---

[5]   More formally stated, $W = \int P \, dV$.

index. It is debatable whether the tension-time index predicts myocardial oxygen consumption with any more certainty than the simple pressure-rate product. The quest for a reliable index of myocardial oxygen consumption continues as cardiac imaging techniques (described near the end of this chapter) make cardiac volume and dimension information more routinely available. For example, this additional information makes it possible to construct ventricular pressure-volume loops whose area accurately indicates external cardiac work. As yet, however, no simple method has been found for assessing all the factors that affect myocardial energy use and using them to predict myocardial oxygen consumption.

MEASUREMENT OF CARDIAC FUNCTION
Cardiac Output/Cardiac Index

Establishing the *absolute* value of a patient's cardiac output is a relatively difficult task. It is, however, possible to estimate the *relative change* in a patient's cardiac output between two situations from the changes in heart rate (HR) and arterial pressure that occur. Recall (from Fig. 4-1) that arterial pulse pressure (P_p) is defined as the difference between the arterial systolic (P_s) and diastolic (P_d) pressures. For reasons that will be explained in Chap. 7, acute changes in pulse pressure occur primarily because of changes in stroke volume (SV). If one assumes a linear relationship between changes in stroke volume and pulse pressure, then one can reason that since $CO = HR \times SV$ the fractional change in CO that occurs in going from situation 1 to situation 2 is approximately equal to the product of the fractional changes in HR and P_p between these situations. For example, if heart rate increased by 10 percent and pulse pressure increased by 10 percent, one would estimate that cardiac output increased by 21 percent (1.1 $\times$ 1.1 = 1.21). (See also Study Question 34.)

There are a number of clinical methods of measuring absolute values of cardiac output that use the Fick principle discussed in Chap. 1. For calculating blood flow, the Fick equation can be rearranged as follows:

$$\dot{Q} = \frac{\dot{X}_{tc}}{[X]_a - [X]_v}$$

A common method of determining cardiac output is to use the Fick principle to calculate the collective flow through the systemic organs from (1) the whole body oxygen consumption rate $(\dot{X}_{tc})$, (2) the oxygen concentration in arterial blood $([X]_a)$, and (3) the concentration of oxygen in mixed venous blood $([X]_v)$. Of the values required for this calculation, the oxygen content of mixed venous blood is the most difficult to obtain. Generally, the sample for venous blood oxygen measurement must be taken from venous catheters positioned in the right ventricle or pulmonary artery to ensure that it is a mixed sample of venous blood from all systemic organs.

The calculation of cardiac output from the Fick principle is best illustrated by an example. Suppose a patient is consuming 250 ml of O_2 per minute when his or her systemic arterial blood contains 200 ml of O_2 per liter and the right ventricular blood contains 150 ml of O_2 per liter. This means that, on the average, each liter of blood loses 50 ml of O_2 as it passes through the systemic organs. In order for 250 ml of O_2 to be consumed per minute, 5 liters of blood must pass through the systemic circulation each minute:

$$\dot{Q} = \frac{250 \text{ ml } O_2/\text{min}}{(200 - 150) \text{ ml } O_2/\text{liter blood}}$$

$$\dot{Q} = 5 \text{ liters blood/min}$$

Dye dilution and thermal dilution (dilution of heat) are other clinical techniques commonly employed for estimating cardiac output. Usually a known quantity of indicator (dye or heat) is rapidly injected into the blood as it enters the right heart and appropriate detectors are arranged to continuously record the concentration of the indicator in blood as it leaves the left heart. It is possible to estimate the cardiac output from the quantity of indicator injected and the time record of indicator concentration in the blood that leaves the left heart.

A typical dye-dilution record is shown in Fig. 4-11. Shortly after the injection of dye into the right heart, the dye concentration in the arterial blood rises to a peak and then begins to decline. A complicating secondary rise in dye concentration occurs as the dye begins to recirculate through the heart. The downslope of the primary peak, however, can be extrapolated (on a semilogarithmic plot) to the abscissa in order to obtain a "single passage" time-concentration curve for the dye. The area under this curve divided by its duration gives the average dye concentration in the arterial blood over this time period. If no dye is lost in the lungs, this average dye concentration must equal the amount of dye injected divided by the volume of blood that came out of the left heart during this time period. Thus it

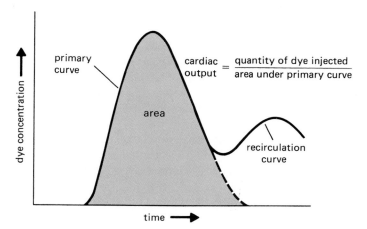

Figure 4-11 Typical dye-dilution curve used to determine cardiac output.

follows that the cardiac output can be calculated by dividing the quantity of dye injected by the area under the primary (single passage) curve of the dye-dilution record. The larger the area under the curve, the less is the cardiac output.

The normal cardiac output for an individual is obviously dependent on his or her size. For example, the cardiac output of 50-kg woman will be significantly lower than that of a 90-kg man. It has been found, however, that cardiac output correlates better with body surface area than body weight. Therefore, it is common to express the cardiac output per square meter of surface area This value is called the *cardiac index;* at rest it is normally approximately 3 (liters/min)/m^2.

Imaging Techniques

Advances in several techniques have made it possible to obtain two- and even three-dimensional images of the heart throughout the cardiac cycle. Visual or computer-aided analysis of such images provides new types of information useful in clinically evaluating cardiac function. These techniques are especially suited for detecting abnormal operation of cardiac valves or contractile function in portions of the heart walls. They also can provide estimates of heart chamber volumes at different times in the cardiac cycle which, as described later, are used in a number of ways to assess cardiac function.

Echocardiography is the most widely used of the three cardiac imaging techniques currently available. This noninvasive technique is based on the fact that a portion of a sound wave reflects back toward the source when it encounters abrupt changes in the density of the medium through which it is traveling. A transducer, placed at specified locations on the chest, generates pulses of ultrasonic waves and detects reflected waves that bounce off the cardiac tissue interfaces. The longer the time between the transmission of the wave and the arrival of the reflection, the deeper the structure is in the thorax. Such information can be reconstructed by computer in various ways to produce a continuous image of the heart and its chambers throughout the cardiac cycle. *Cardiac angiography* involves the placement of catheters into the right or left ventricle and injection of radiopaque contrast medium during high speed x-ray filming (cineradiography). *Radionuclide ventriculography* involves the intravenous injection of a radioactive isotope that stays in the vascular space (usually technitium that binds to red blood cells) and the measurement of the changes in intensity of radiation detected over the ventricles during the cardiac cycle.

Cardiac Contractility Estimates   The information derived from these imaging techniques is being used for evaluating myocardial contractility, a critically important parameter of cardiac function that has been difficult to measure in a clinical setting.

Ejection fraction is defined as the ratio of stroke volume (SV) to end-diastolic volume (EDV):

EF = SV/EDV

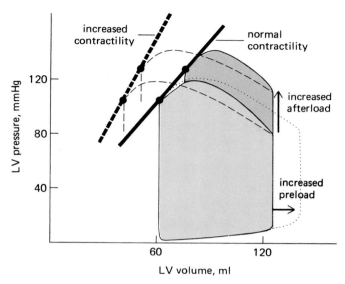

Figure 4-12   The effect of increased contractility upon the LV end-systolic pressure-volume relationship.

Ejection fraction is commonly expressed as a percentage and normally ranges
from 55 to 80 percent (mean 67 percent) under resting conditions. Ejection frac-
tions of less than 55 percent indicate depressed myocardial contractility.

The imaging techniques can also be used to determine the *end-systolic pressure-volume relationship* (see Fig. 4-7*B*). End-systolic volume for a given cardiac
cycle is estimated by one of the imaging techniques described above while end-
systolic pressure for that cardiac cycle is obtained from the arterial pressure
record at the point of the closure of the aortic valve (the incisura). Values for several different cardiac cycles are obtained during infusion of a vasoconstrictor
(which alters afterload), and the data are plotted. As shown in Fig. 4-12, increases
in myocardial contractility are associated with an upward shift in this relationship. Decreases in contractility (as may be caused by heart disease) are associated
with a downward shift of the line and will be discussed further in Chap. 12. This
method of assessing cardiac function is particularly important because it provides
an estimate of contractility that is independent of the end-diastolic volume (preload). Recall from Fig. 4-6 and from the pressure-volume loop described by the
dotted line in Fig. 4-12 that increases in preload cause increases in stroke volume
without changing the end-systolic volume. Thus only alterations in contractility
will cause shifts in the end-systolic pressure-volume relationship.

Study Questions: 11 to 16

5

THE ELECTROCARDIOGRAM

OBJECTIVES

The student understands the physiological basis of the electrocardiogram:

1 States the relationship between electrical events of cardiac excitation and the P, QRS, and T waves, the PR interval, and the ST segment of the electrocardiogram.
2 States Einthoven's basic electrocardiographic conventions and, given data, determines the mean electrical axis of the heart.
3 Describes the standard 12-lead electrocardiogram.

BASIC FEATURES OF THE ELECTROCARDIOGRAM

A typical electrocardiographic record is indicated in Fig. 5-1. As briefly described in Chap. 3, the major features of the electrocardiogram are the P, QRS, and T waves which are caused by atrial depolarization, ventricular depolarization, and ventricular repolarization, respectively. The period of time from the initiation of the P wave to the beginning of QRS complex is designated as the PR interval and indicates the time it takes for an action potential to spread through the atria and the atrioventricular (AV) node. During the later portion of the PR interval (PR segment), no voltages are detected on the body surface. This is because atrial muscle cells are depolarized (in the plateau phase of their action potentials), ventricular cells are still resting, and the electrical field set up by the action potential progressing through the small AV node is not intense enough to be detected. The duration of the normal PR interval ranges from 120 to 200 ms. Shortly after the cardiac impulse breaks out of the AV node and into the rapidly conducting Purkinje system, all the ventricular muscle cells depolarize within a very short period of time and cause the QRS complex. The R wave is the largest event in the electrocardiogram because ventricular muscle cells are so numerous and because they depolarize nearly in unison. The normal QRS complex lasts between 60 and 100 ms. [The repolarization of atrial cells is also occurring during the time period in which ventricular depolarization generates the QRS complex on the electrocardiogram (see Fig. 3-5). Atrial repolarization is not evident on the electrocardiogram because it is a poorly synchronized event in a relatively

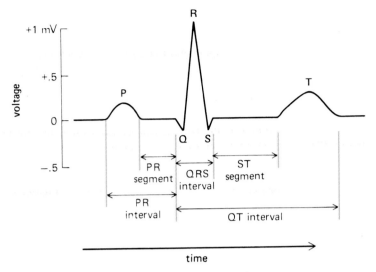

Figure 5-1   Typical electrocardiogram.

small mass of heart tissue that is completely overshadowed by the major events occurring in the ventricles at this time.]

The QRS complex is followed by the *ST segment.* Normally, no electrical potentials are measured on the body surface during the ST segment because no rapid changes in membrane potential are occurring in any of the cells of the heart; atrial cells have already returned to the resting phase, whereas ventricular muscle cells are in the plateau phase of their action potentials. (Myocardial injury or inadequate blood flow, however, can produce elevations or depressions in the ST segment.) When ventricular cells begin to repolarize, a voltage once again appears on the body surface and is measured as the T wave of the electrocardiogram. The T wave is broader and not as large as the R wave because ventricular repolarization is less synchronous than depolarization. At the conclusion of the T wave all the cells in the heart are in the resting state. No body surface potential is measured until the next impulse is generated by the sinoatrial (SA) node.

It should be recognized that the operation of the specialized conduction system is a primary factor in determining the normal electrocardiographic pattern. For example, the AV nodal transmission time determines the PR interval. Also, the effectiveness of the Purkinje system in synchronizing ventricular depolarization is reflected in the large magnitude and short duration of the QRS complex. it should also be noted that nearly every heart muscle cell is inherently capable of rhythmicity and that all cardiac cells are electrically interconnected through gap junctions. Thus a functional heart rhythm can and often does occur without the involvement of part or all of the specialized conduction system. Such a situation is, however, abnormal, and the existence of abnormal conduction pathways would produce an abnormal electrocardiogram.

Basic Electrocardiographic Conventions

Recording electrocardiograms has become a routine diagnostic procedure, which has been standardized by universal application of certain conventions. The conventions for recording and analysis of electrocardiograms from the three standard bipolar limb leads are briefly described here.

Recording electrodes are placed on both arms and the left leg—usually at the wrists and ankle. The assumptions are made that the appendages act merely as extensions of the recording system and that voltage measurements are made between points that form an equilateral triangle over the thorax, as shown in Fig. 5-2. This conceptualization is called *Einthoven's triangle* in honor of the Dutch physiologist who devised it at the turn of the century. Any single electrocardiographic trace is recording of the voltage difference measured between any two vertices of Einthoven's triangle. We have already shown an example of the lead II electrocardiogram measured between the right arm and the left leg (Fig. 5-1). Similarly, lead I and lead III electrocardiograms represent voltage measurements taken along the other two sides of Einthoven's triangle, as indicated in Fig. 5-2. The + and − symbols in Fig. 5-2 indicate polarity conventions that have been universally adopted. For example, an upward deflection in a lead II electrocardiogram (as normally occurs during the P, R, and T waves) indicates that the voltage measured at the left leg is more positive than that at the right shoulder. Similar polarity conventions have been established for lead I and lead III recordings and are indicated by the + and − symbols in Fig. 5-2. In addition, electrocardiographic recording equipment is often standardized so that 1 cm on

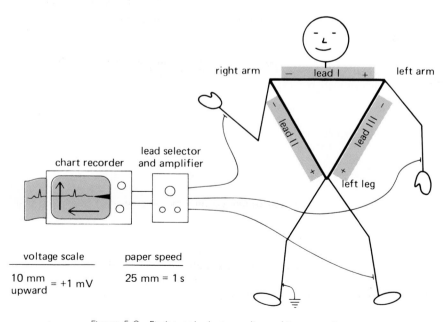

Figure 5-2   Einthoven's electrocardiographic conventions.

the vertical axis always represents a potential difference of 1 mV, and that 25 mm on the horizontal axis of any electrocardiographic record represents 1 s. Most electrocardiographic records contain calibration signals so that abnormal rates and wave amplitudes can be easily detected.

As shown later in this chapter, many cardiac electrical abnormalities can be detected in recordings from a single electrocardiographic lead. However, certain clinically useful information must be derived by combining the information obtained from two electrocardiographic leads. To understand these more complex electrocardiographic analyses, we must first examine more closely how voltages appear on the body surface as a result of the cardiac electrical activity.

CARDIAC DIPOLES AND ELECTROCARDIOGRAPHIC RECORDS

Einthoven's conceptualization of how cardiac electrical activity causes potential differences on the surface of the body is illustrated in Fig. 5-3. In this example, the heart is shown at one instant in the atrial depolarization phase. The cardiac impulse, after having arisen in the SA node, is spreading as a wavefront of depolarization through the atrial tissue. At each point along this wavefront of electrical activity, a small charge separation exists between polarized membranes (positive outside) and depolarized membranes (negative outside). Thus the wavefront may be thought of as a series of individual *electrical dipoles* (regions of charge separation). Each individual dipole is oriented in the direction of local wavefront movement. The large black arrow in Fig. 5-3 represents the total net dipole created by the summed contributions of all the individual dipoles distributed along the wavefront of depolarization. The net dipole which exists at any instant is oriented (i.e., points) in the general direction of wavefront movement at that instant. The magnitude or strength of the dipole (represented here by the arrow length) is determined by: (1) how extensive the wavefront is (i.e., how many

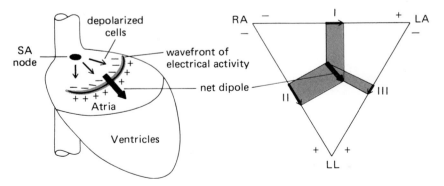

Figure 5-3   Net cardiac dipole during atrial depolarization and its components on the limb leads.

cells are simultaneously depolarizing at the instant in question) and (2) the consistency of orientation between individual dipoles at different points in the wavefront (dipoles with the same orientation reinforce each other; dipoles with opposite orientation tend to cancel each other).

The net dipole in the example of Fig. 5-3 causes the lower-left portion of the body to be generally positive with respect to the upper-right portion. This particular dipole will cause positive voltages to exist on all three of the electrocardiogram limb leads. As shown in the right half of Fig. 5-3, this can be deduced from Einthoven's triangle by observing that the net dipole has some component which points in the positive direction of leads I, II, and III. As illustrated in Fig. 5-3, the component which a cardiac dipole has on a given electrocardiogram lead is found by drawing perpendicular lines from the appropriate side of Einthoven's triangle to the tip and tail of the dipole. (It may be helpful to think of the component on each lead as the "shadow" cast by the dipole on that lead as a result of a "sun" located far beyond the corner of Einthoven's triangle that is opposite the lead.) Note that the dipole in this example is most parallel to lead II and therefore has a large component in the lead II direction. Thus it will create a larger voltage on lead II than on leads I or III. This dipole has a rather small component on lead III because it is oriented nearly perpendicular to lead III.

The limb lead configuration may be thought of as a way to view the heart's electrical activity from three different perspectives (or axes). The vector representing the heart's instantaneous dipole strength and orientation is the object under observation, and its appearance depends on the position from which it is viewed. The instantaneous voltage measured on the axis of lead I, for example, indicates how the dipole being generated by the heart's electrical activity at that instant appears when viewed from directly above. A cardiac dipole that is oriented horizontally appears large on lead I, whereas a vertically oriented cardiac dipole, however large, produces no voltage on lead I. Thus it is necessary to have views from two directions to establish the magnitude and orientation of the heart's dipole. A vertically oriented dipole would be invisible on lead I but would be readily apparent if viewed from the perspective of lead II or lead III.

It is important to recognize that the example of Fig. 5-3 pertains only to one instant during atrial depolarization. The net cardiac dipole continually changes in magnitude and orientation during the course of atrial depolarization. The nature of these changes will determine the shape of the P wave on each of the electrocardiogram leads.

The P wave terminates when the wave of depolarization, as illustrated in Fig. 5-3, reaches the nonmuscular border between the atria and the ventricles and the number of individual dipoles becomes very small. At this time, the cardiac impulse is still being slowly transmitted toward the ventricles through the AV node. However, the electrical activity in the AV node involves so few cells that it generates no detectable net cardiac dipole. Thus, no voltages are measured on the surface of the body for a brief period following the P wave. A net cardiac dipole reappears only when the depolarization completes its passage through the AV node, enters the Purkinje system, and begins its rapid passage through the ventricular muscle cells. Because the Purkinje fibers terminate in the intraventricular septum and in the endocardial layers at the apex of the ventricles, ventricular depolarization occurs first in these areas and then proceeds outward and upward through the ventricular myocardium.

Ventricular Depolarization and the QRS Complex

It is the rapid and large changes in the magnitude and direction of the net cardiac dipole that exist during ventricular depolarization which cause the QRS complex of the electrocardiogram. The normal process is illustrated in Fig. 5-4. The initial ventricular depolarization usually occurs on the left side of the intraventricular septum as diagramed in the upper panel of the figure. Analysis of the cardiac dipole formed by this initial ventricular depolarization with the aid of Einthoven's triangle shows that this dipole has a negative component on lead I, a small negative component on lead II, and a positive component on lead III. The upper right panel shows the actual deflections on each of the electrocardiographic limb leads which will be produced by this dipole. Note that it is possible for a given cardiac dipole to produce opposite deflections on different leads.

The second row of panels in Fig. 5-4 shows the ventricles during the instant in ventricular depolarization when the number of individual dipoles is greatest and/or their orientation is most similar. This phase generates the large net cardiac dipole which is responsible for the R wave of the electrocardiogram. In Fig. 5-4, the net cardiac dipole is nearly parallel to lead II. As indicated, such a dipole produces large positive R waves on all three limbs leads.

The third row of diagrams in Fig. 5-4 shows the situation near the end of the spread of depolarization through the ventricles and indicates how the small net cardiac dipole present at this time produces the S wave. Note that an S wave does not necessarily appear on all electrocardiogram leads (as in lead I of this example).

The bottom row of diagrams in Fig. 5-4 shows that during the ST segment, all ventricular muscle cells are in a depolarized state. There are no waves of electrical activity moving through the heart tissue. Consequently, no net cardiac dipole exists at this time and no voltage differences exist between points on the body surface. All electrocardiographic traces will be flat at the *isoelectric* (zero voltage) level.

Ventricular Repolarization and the T Wave

As illustrated in Fig. 5-1, the T wave is normally positive on lead II as is the R wave. This indicates that the net cardiac dipole generated during ventricular repolarization is oriented in the same general direction as that which exists during ventricular depolarization. This is somewhat surprising since the individual dipoles generated along a wave front of repolarization have exactly the opposite polarity as those which exist along a wave front of depolarization. However, recall from Fig. 3-5 that the last ventricular cells to depolarize are the first to repo-

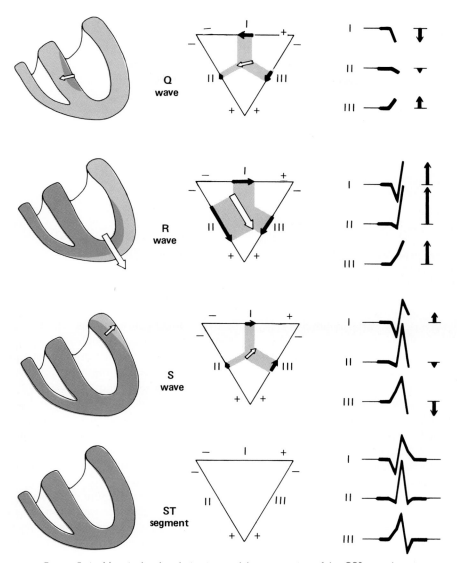

Figure 5-4   Ventricular depolarization and the generation of the QRS complex.

larize. The reasons for this are not well understood but the result is that the wave front of electrical activity during ventricular repolarization tends to retrace, in *reverse direction,* the course followed during ventricular depolarization. The product of reversed individual dipole polarity and reversed wave front propagation pathway during ventricular repolarization is a positive T wave. The T wave is broader and smaller than the R wave because the repolarization of ventricular cells is less well synchronized than is their depolarization.

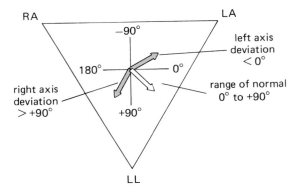

Figure 5-5 Mean electrical axis and axis deviations.

MEAN ELECTRICAL AXIS AND AXIS DEVIATIONS

The orientation of the cardiac dipole during the most intense phase of ventricular depolarization (i.e., at the instant the R wave reaches its peak) is called the *mean electrical axis* of the heart. It is used clinically as an indicator of whether or not ventricular depolarization is proceeding over normal pathways. The mean electrical axis is reported in degrees according to the convention indicated in Fig. 5-5. (Note that the downward direction corresponds to *plus* 90° in this system.) As indicated, a mean electrical axis which lies anywhere in the patient's lower left-hand quadrant is considered normal. A *left axis deviation* exists when the mean electrical axis falls in the patient's upper left-hand quadrant and may indicate a physical displacement of the heart to the left, left ventricular hypertrophy, or loss of electrical activity in the right ventricle. A *right axis deviation* exists when the mean electrical axis falls in the patient's lower right-hand quadrant and may indicate a physical displacement of the heart to the right, right ventricular hypertrophy, or loss of electrical activity in the left ventricle.

The mean electrical axis of the heart can be determined from electrocardiograms recorded on any two leads by reversing the process that was illustrated in Fig. 5-4. The steps to follow include: (1) measuring the magnitude of the R waves on the two records,[1] (2) plotting these magnitudes as components on the appropriate sides of Einthoven's equilateral triangle according to the standardized polarity conventions, (3) projecting perpendicular lines from the heads and tails of these components into the interior of the triangle to find the position of the head and tail of the cardiac dipole which produced the R waves, and (4) measuring the angular orientation of this dipole. An approximate short-cut method is to scan the electrocardiogram records for the lead tracing with the largest R waves and then to deduce that the mean electrical axis must be nearly parallel to that lead. In Fig. 5-4, for example, the largest R wave occurs on lead II. Lead II has an orientation of + 60° which is very close to the actual mean electrical axis in this example.

---

[1] For reasons that are beyond the scope of this text, it is somewhat more appropriate to use the algebraic sum of the R and S wave magnitudes.

Another analysis technique called *vectorcardiography* is based on continuously following the magnitude and orientation of the heart's dipole throughout the cardiac cycle. A typical vectorcardiogram is illustrated in Fig. 5-6. If one imagines the heart's electrical dipole as a vector with its tail always positioned at the center of Einthoven's triangle, then the vectorcardiogram can be thought of as a complete record of all the various positions that the head of the dipole assumes during the course of one cardiac cycle. A vectorcardiogram starts from an isoelectric diastolic point and traces three loops during each cardiac cycle. The first small loop is caused by atrial depolarization, the second large loop is caused by ventricular depolarization, and the final intermediate-sized loop is caused by ventricular repolarization. The mean electrical axis of the heart is immediately apparent in a vectorcardiographic reading.

THE STANDARD 12-LEAD ELECTROCARDIOGRAM

The standard clinical electrocardiogram involves voltage measurements recorded from 12 different leads. Three of these are the bipolar limb leads I, II, and III which we have already discussed.

It is also possible, however, to record electrical potentials generated by the heart in a unipolar fashion. In this situation, two of the limb electrodes are electrically connected to form an *indifferent electrode* while the third limb electrode is made the positive pole of the pair. Recordings made from these electrodes are called *augmented unipolar limb leads.* The voltage record obtained between the electrode at the right arm and the indifferent electrode is called a lead aVR electrocardiogram. Similarly, lead aVL is recorded from the electrode on the left arm and lead aVF is recorded from the electrode on the left leg.

The standard limb leads (I, II, and III) and the augmented unipolar limb leads (aVR, aVL, and aVF) record the electrical activity of the heart as it appears from six different "perspectives," all in the frontal plane. As shown in Fig. 5-7A, the axes for leads I, II, and III are those of the sides of Einthoven's

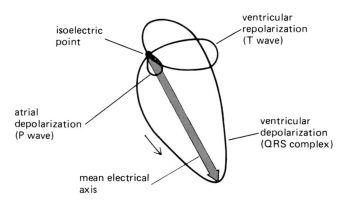

Figure 5-6 Typical vectorcardiogram.

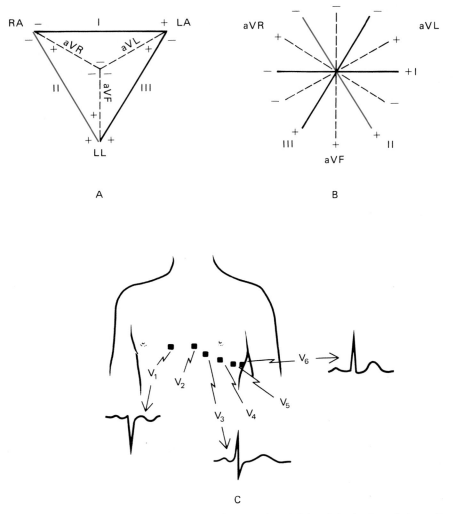

Figure 5-7   The standard 12-lead electrocardiogram. A and B. Leads in the frontal plane. C. Electrode positions for precordial leads in the transverse plane.

triangle, while those for aVR, aVL and aVF are specified by lines drawn from the center of Einthoven's triangle to each of its vertices. As indicated in Fig. 5-7B, the six limb leads can be thought of as a hexaxial reference system for observing the cardiac vectors in the frontal plane.

The other six leads of the standard 12-lead electrocardiogram are also unipolar leads which "look" at the electrical vector projections in the transverse plane. These potentials are obtained by placing an additional (*exploring*) electrode in six specified positions on the chest wall as shown in Fig. 5-7C. The indifferent electrode in this case is formed by electrically connecting the limb electrodes. These leads are identified as *precordial* or *chest* leads and are designated as V1 through V6. As shown in this figure, when the positive electrode is placed in position 1 and the wave of ventricular excitation sweeps away from it, the resultant deflection will be downward. When the electrode is in position 6 and the wave of ventricular excitation sweeps toward it, the deflection will be upward.

Study Questions: 17 and 18

6

CARDIAC ABNORMALITIES

OBJECTIVES

The student, through understanding normal cardiac function, diagnoses and appreciates the consequences of common cardiac abnormalities:

1 Detects common cardiac arrhythmias from the electrocardiogram, identifies their physiological bases, and describes their physiological consequences.
2 Lists four common valvular abnormalities for the left heart and describes the alterations in heart sounds and intracardiac pressure and flow patterns that accompany them.

Recall that effective, efficient ventricular pumping action depends on proper cardiac function in five basic respects (see p. 19). In this chapter, we shall focus on abnormalities in three of these respects: (1) abnormal cardiac excitation and rhythmicity, (2) valvular stenosis (inadequate valve opening), and (3) valvular insufficiency (incomplete valve closure). Discussion of abnormalities in myocardial force production and cardiac filling will be presented in later chapters.

ELECTRICAL ABNORMALITIES AND ARRHYTHMIAS

Many cardiac excitation problems can be diagnosed from the information in a single lead of an electrocardiogram, as illustrated in Fig. 6-1. The lead II electrocardiogram trace at the top of this figure is identified as normal sinus rhythm based on the following characteristics: (1) the frequency of QRS complexes are ~ 1 per second indicating a normal rate, (2) the shape of the QRS complex is normal for lead II and its duration is less than 120 ms indicating rapid depolarization of the ventricles via normal conduction pathways, (3) each QRS complex is preceded by a P wave of proper configuration indicating sinoatrial (SA) nodal origin of the excitation, (4) the PR interval is less than 200 ms indicating proper conduction delay of the impulse spread through the atrioventricular (AV) node, and (5) there are no extra P waves indicating that no AV nodal conduction block is present. The subsequent EKG tracings in Fig. 6-1 represent irregularities commonly found in clinical practice. Examination of each of these traces with the above characteristics in mind will aid in the differential diagnosis.

Supraventricular tachycardia (sometimes called paroxysmal atrial tachycardia) occurs when the atria are abnormally excited and drive the ventricles at a very rapid rate. These paroxysms begin abruptly, last for a few minutes to a few hours, and then, just as abruptly, disappear and heart rate reverts to normal. QRS complexes appear normal (albeit frequent) with simple paroxysmal atrial tachycardia because the ventricular conduction pathways operate normally. The P and T waves may be superimposed because of the high heart rate. Low blood pressure and fainting may accompany bouts of this arrhythmia because the extremely high heart rate does not allow sufficient diastolic time for ventricular filling.

There are two mechanisms that may account for this abnormality. First, an atrial region, usually outside the SA node, may become irritable (perhaps because of local interruption in blood flow) and begin to fire rapidly to take over the pacemaker function. Such an abnormal pacemaker region is called an *ectopic*

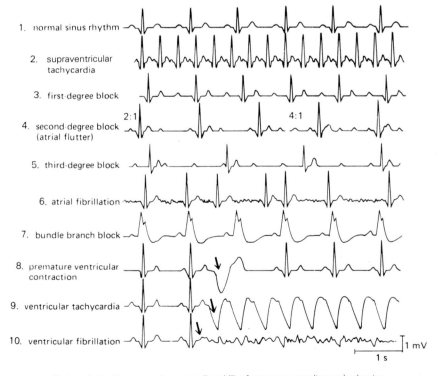

Figure 6-1   Electrocardiograms (lead II) of common cardiac arrhythmias.

focus. Alternatively, atrial conduction may become altered so that a single wave of excitation does not die out but continually travels around some abnormal atrial conduction loop. In this case the continual activity in the conduction loop may drive the atria and AV node at a very high frequency. This self-sustaining process is called a *reentry phenomenon* and is diagramed in Fig. 6-2. This situation may develop as a result of abnormal repolarization and altered refractory periods in local areas of the myocardium.

In *first-degree heart block* (shown in trace 3 of Fig. 6-1), the only electrical abnormality is unusually slow conduction through the AV node. This condition is detected by an abnormally long PR interval (> 0.2 s). Otherwise, the electrocardiogram may be completely normal. At normal heart rates the physiological effects of a first-degree block are inconsequential.

A *second-degree heart block* (trace 4 of Fig. 6-1) is said to exist when some but not all atrial impulses are transmitted through the AV node to the ventricle. Impulses are blocked in the AV node if the cells of the region are still in a refractory period from a previous excitation. The situation is aggravated by high atrial rates and slower than normal conduction through the AV nodal region. In second-degree block, some but not all P waves are accompanied by corresponding QRS complexes and T waves. Atrial rate is often faster than ventricular rate by a certain ratio (e.g., $2:1$, $3:1$, $4:1$). This condition may not represent a serious clinical problem as long as the ventricular rate is adequate to meet the pumping needs. The term *atrial flutter* is often applied when very high atrial rates occur and are not accompanied by high ventricular rates.

In *third-degree heart block* (trace 5 of Fig. 6-1), no impulses are transmitted through the AV node. Some area in the ventricles—often in the common bundle or bundle branches near the exit of the AV node—assumes the pacemaker role for the ventricular tissue. Atrial rate and ventricular rate are completely independent, and P waves and QRS complexes are totally dissociated in the electrocardiogram. Ventricular rate is likely to be slower than normal (bradycardia) and sometimes is slow enough to impair cardiac output.

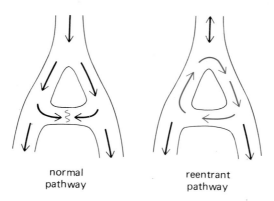

normal
pathway

reentrant
pathway

Figure 6-2   Normal and reentrant cardiac excitation pathways.

Atrial fibrillation (trace 6 of Fig. 6-1) is characterized by a complete loss of the normally close synchrony of the excitation and resting phases between individual atrial cells. Cells in different areas of the atria depolarize, repolarize, and are excited again randomly. Consequently, no P waves appear in the electrocardiogram although there may be rapid irregular small waves apparent throughout diastole. The ventricular rate is often very irregular in atrial fibrillation because impulses enter the AV node from the atria at unpredictable times. Fibrillation is a self-sustaining process. The mechanisms behind it are not well understood, but impulses are thought to progress repeatedly around irregular conduction pathways (sometimes called circus pathways which imply a reentry phenomenon as described earlier and in Fig. 6-2). However, because atrial contraction usually plays a negligible role in ventricular filling, atrial fibrillation is generally tolerated by most patients as long as ventricular rate is sufficient to maintain the cardiac output.

Conduction blocks called *bundle branch blocks* or *hemiblocks* (trace 7 of Fig. 6-1) can occur in either of the branches of the Purkinje system of the intraventricular septum often as a result of a myocardial infarction. Depolarization is less synchronous than normal in the half of the heart with the nonfunctional Purkinje system. This results in a widening of the QRS complex (> 0.12 s) because a longer time is required for ventricular depolarization to be completed (0.12 s is the usual normal upper limit). The physiological effects of bundle branch blocks are usually inconsequential.

Premature ventricular contractions (trace 8 of Fig. 6-1) are caused by action potentials initiated by and propagated away from an ectopic focus in the ventricle. As a result, the ventricle depolarizes and contracts before it normally would. A premature ventricular contraction is often followed by a missed beat (called a *compensatory pause*) because the ventricular cells are still refractory when the next normal impulse emerges from the SA node. The highly abnormal ventricular depolarization pattern of a premature ventricular contraction produces the large-amplitude, long-duration deflections on the electrocardiogram. The shapes of the electrocardiographic records of these extra beats are highly variable and depend on the ectopic site of their origin and the depolarization pathways involved. The volume of blood ejected by the premature beat itself is smaller than normal, whereas the stroke volume of the beat following the compensatory pause is larger than normal. This is due partly to the differences in filling times and partly to an inherent phenomenon of cardiac muscle called *postextrasystolic potentiation.* Single premature ventricular contractions (PVC) occur occasionally in most individuals and, although sometimes alarming to the individual experiencing them, are not dangerous. Frequent occurrence of PVCs, however, may be a signal of possible myocardial damage.

Ventricular tachycardia (trace 9 of Fig. 6-1) occurs when the ventricles are driven at high rates by impulses originating from ventricular ectopic foci. Ventricular tachycardia is a very serious condition. Not only is diastolic filling time limited by the rapid rate, but the abnormal excitation pathways make ventricular contraction less synchronous and therefore less effective than normal. In addition, ventricular tachycardia often precedes ventricular fibrillation.

In *ventricular fibrillation* (trace 10 of Fig. 6-1), various areas of the ventricle are excited and contract asynchronously. The mechanisms are similar to those in atrial fibrillation. The ventricle is especially susceptible to fibrillation whenever a premature excitation occurs at the end of the T wave of the previous excitation, i.e., when most ventricular cells are in the "hyperexcitable" or "vulnerable" period of their electrical cycle. In addition, because some cells are repolarized and some are still refractory, circus pathways can be triggered easily at this time. Since no pumping action occurs with ventricular fibrillation, the situation is fatal unless quickly corrected by cardiac conversion. During conversion, the artificial application of large currents to the entire heart may be effective in depolarizing all heart cells simultaneously and thus allowing a normal excitation pathway to be reestablished.

VALVULAR ABNORMALITIES

Pumping action of the heart is impaired when the valves do not function properly. Abnormal heart sounds, which usually accompany cardiac valvular defects, are called *murmurs*. These sounds are caused by abnormal pressure gradients and turbulent blood flow patterns that occur during the cardiac cycle. A number of techniques, ranging from simple auscultation (listening to the heart sounds) to echocardiography or cardiac catheterization, are used to obtain information about the nature and extent of the malfunction. A brief overview of four of the common valve defects is given in Fig. 6-3.

Some consequences of *aortic stenosis* are shown in Fig. 6-3*A*. Normally, the aortic valve represents a pathway of very low resistance through which blood leaves the left ventricle. If this opening is narrowed (stenotic), its resistance increases. A significant pressure difference between the left ventricle and the aorta may be required to eject blood through a stenotic aortic valve. As shown in Fig. 6-3*A*, intraventricular pressures may rise to very high levels during systole while aortic pressure rises more slowly than normal to a systolic value that is subnormal. Pulse pressure is usually low with aortic stenosis. High intraventricular pressure development is a strong stimulus for cardiac muscle cell hypertrophy, and an increase in left ventricular muscle mass invariably accompanies aortic stenosis. This tends to produce a leftward deviation of the electrical axis. (The mean electrical axis will fall in the upper right-hand quadrant of the diagram in Fig. 5-5) Blood being ejected through the narrowed orifice may reach very high velocities, and turbulent flow may occur in the aorta. This abnormal turbulent flow can be heard as a *systolic* (or ejection) *murmur* with a properly placed stethoscope.

Some consequences of *mitral stenosis* are shown in Fig. 6-3*B*. A pressure difference of more than a few millimeters of mercury across the mitral valve during diastole is distinctly abnormal and indicates that this valve is stenotic. The high resistance mandates an elevated pressure difference to achieve normal flow cross the valve ($Q = \Delta P/R$). Consequently, as shown in Fig. 6-3*B*, left atrial

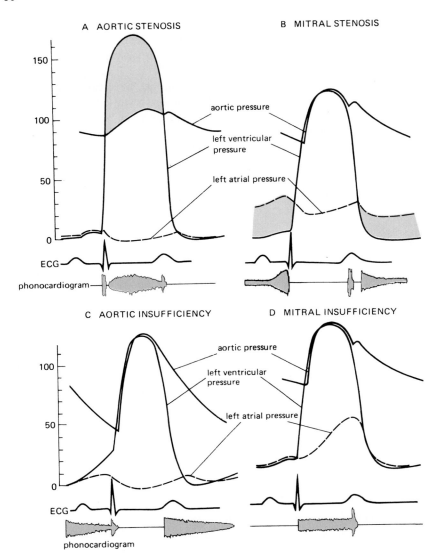

Figure 6-3   Common valvular abnormalities. *A.* Aortic stenosis. *B.* Mitral stenosis. *C.* Aortic regurgitation (insufficiency). *D.* Mitral insufficiency.

pressure and volume are elevated with mitral stenosis. The high left atrial pressure is reflected back into the pulmonary bed and, if high enough, causes "shortness of breath" and pulmonary congestion. A *diastolic murmur* associated with turbulent flow through the stenotic mitral valve can often be heard.

Typical consequences of *aortic regurgitation (insufficiency)* are shown in Fig. 6-3C. When the leaflets of the aortic valve do not provide an adequate seal, blood regurgitates from the aorta back into the left ventricle during the diastolic period. Aortic pressure falls faster and further than normal during diastole, which causes a low diastolic pressure and a large pulse pressure. In addition, ventricular end-diastolic volume and pressure are higher than normal because of the extra blood that reenters the chamber through the incompetent aortic valve during diastole. Turbulent flow of the blood reentering the left ventricle during early diastole produces a characteristic diastolic murmur. Often the aortic valve is altered so that it is both stenotic and insufficient. In these instances both a systolic and a diastolic murmur are present.

Typical consequences of *mitral insufficiency* are shown in Fig. 6-3D. When the mitral valve is insufficient, some blood regurgitates from the left ventricle into the left atrium during systole. A systolic murmur may accompany this abnormal flow pattern. Left atrial pressure is raised to abnormally high levels, and left ventricular end-diastolic volume and pressure increase. Mitral valve *prolapse* is a common form of mitral insufficiency in which the valve leaflets evert into the left atrium during systole.

Study Questions: 19 to 23

7

THE PERIPHERAL VASCULAR SYSTEM

OBJECTIVES

The student understands the physical factors that regulate blood flow through the various components of the vasculature:

1 Lists the major different types of vessels in a vascular bed and describes the morphological differences among them.
2 Given data, calculates the equivalent vascular resistances of networks of vessels arranged in parallel and in series.
3 Describes differences in the blood flow velocity in the various segments and how these differences are related to their total cross-sectional area.
4 Describes laminar and turbulent flow patterns and the origin of flow sounds in the cardiovascular system.
5 Identifies the approximate percentage of the total blood volume that is contained in the various vascular segments in the systemic circulation.
6 Defines a peripheral venous pool and central venous pool.
7 Describes the pressure changes that occur as blood flows through a vascular bed and relates them to the vascular resistance of the various vascular segments.
8 States how the resistance of each consecutive vascular segment contributes to an organ's overall vascular resistance and, given data, calculates the overall resistance.
9 Defines total peripheral resistance and states the relationship between it and the vascular resistance of each systemic organ.
10 Defines vascular compliance and states how the volume-pressure curves for arteries and veins differ.
11 Predicts what will happen to venous volume when venous smooth muscle is activated or venous pressure is changed.
12 Describes the role of arterial compliance in storing energy for blood circulation.
13 Describes how arterial compliance changes with age and how this affects arterial pulse pressure.

14 Describes the auscultation technique of determining arterial systolic and diastolic pressures.

15 Identifies the physical bases of the Korotkoff sounds.

16 Indicates the relationship between arterial pressure, cardiac output, and total peripheral resistance and predicts how arterial pressure will be altered when cardiac output and/or total peripheral resistance change.

17 Given arterial systolic and diastolic pressures, estimates mean arterial pressure.

18 Indicates the relationship between pulse pressure, stroke volume, and arterial compliance and predicts how pulse pressure will be changed by changes in stroke volume, or arterial compliance.

This chapter will describe the overall structural design of the vascular system and discuss the functional implications of this design. Much of this discussion also applies to the pulmonary vascular bed; the main exception is that the pulmonary arterial pressure is much lower than the systemic arterial pressure.

BASIC VASCULAR ARCHITECTURE

Blood that is ejected into the aorta by the left heart passes consecutively through many different types of vessels before it returns to the right heart. As diagramed in Fig. 7-1, the major vessel classifications are *arteries, arterioles, capillaries, venules,* and *veins.* These consecutive vascular segments are distinguished from one another by differences in physical dimensions, morphological characteristics, and function. One thing that all vessels have in common is that they are lined with a contiguous single layer of endothelial cells. In fact, this is true for the entire circulatory system including the heart chamber and even the valve leaflets.

Some representative physical characteristics are shown in Fig. 7-1 for each of the major vessel types. It should be realized, however, that the vascular bed is a continuum and that the transition from one type of vascular segment to another does not occur abruptly. The total cross-sectional area through which blood flows at any particular level in the vascular system is equal to the sum of the cross-sectional areas of all the individual vessels arranged in parallel at that level. The number and total cross-sectional area values presented in Fig. 7-1 are estimates for the entire systemic circulation.

Arteries are thick-walled vessels that contain, in addition to smooth muscle, a large component of elastin and collagen fibers. Primarily because of the elastin fibers, which can stretch to twice their unloaded length, arteries can expand to accept and temporarily store some of the blood ejected by the heart during systole and then, by passive recoil, supply this blood to the organs downstream during diastole. The aorta is the largest artery and has an inside diameter of about 25 mm. Arterial diameter decreases with each consecutive branching, and the smallest arteries have diameters of approximately 0.1 mm. The consecutive arterial branching pattern causes an exponential increase in arterial numbers. Thus, while individual vessels get progressively smaller, the total cross-sectional area

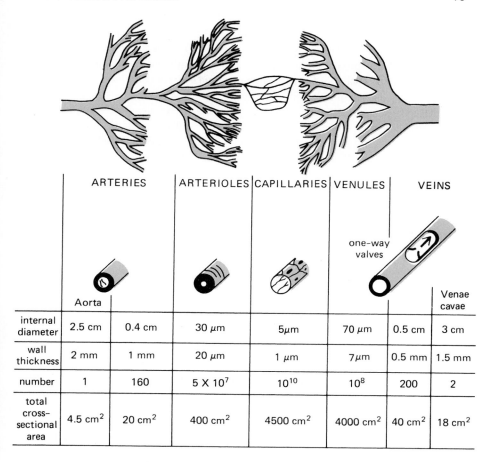

	ARTERIES		ARTERIOLES	CAPILLARIES	VENULES	VEINS	
	Aorta				one-way valves		Venae cavae
internal diameter	2.5 cm	0.4 cm	30 μm	5μm	70 μm	0.5 cm	3 cm
wall thickness	2 mm	1 mm	20 μm	1 μm	7μm	0.5 mm	1.5 mm
number	1	160	5×10^7	10^{10}	10^8	200	2
total cross-sectional area	4.5 cm^2	20 cm^2	400 cm^2	4500 cm^2	4000 cm^2	40 cm^2	18 cm^2

Figure 7-1   Structural characteristics of the peripheral vascular system.

available for blood flow within the arterial system increases to severalfold that in the aorta.

Arterioles are smaller and structured differently than arteries. In proportion to lumen size, arterioles have much thicker walls with more smooth muscle and less elastic material than arteries. Because arterioles are so muscular, their diameters can be actively changed to regulate the blood flow through peripheral organs. Despite their minute size, arterioles are so numerous that in parallel their collective cross-sectional area is much larger than that at any level in arteries.

Capillaries are the smallest vessels in the vasculature. In fact, red blood cells with diameters of 7 μm must deform to pass through them. As discussed in Chap. 1, the capillary wall consists of a single layer of endothelial cells, which separate the blood from the interstitial fluid by only about 1 μm. Capillaries contain no smooth muscle and thus lack the ability to change their diameters actively. They are so numerous that the total collective cross-sectional area of all the capillaries in systemic organs is more than 1000 times that of the root of the aorta. Given that capillaries are about 0.5 mm in length, we can calculate that the total surface area available for exchange of material between blood and interstitial fluid exceeds 100 m^2.

After leaving capillaries, blood is collected in venules and veins and returned to the heart. Venous vessels have very thin walls in proportion to their diameters. Their walls contain smooth muscle and the diameters of venous vessels can actively change. Because of their thin walls, venous vessels are quite distensible. Therefore, their diameters change passively in response to small changes in transmural distending pressure, which is the difference between the internal and external pressures. Venous vessels, especially the larger ones, also have one-way valves that prevent reverse flow. As we shall see later, these valves are especially important in the cardiovascular system's operation during standing and during exercise.

BASIC VASCULAR FUNCTION

Resistance and Flow in Networks of Vessels

The basic flow equation $(\dot{Q} = \Delta P/R)$ may be applied to networks of tubes by the same rules with which an analogous equation, Ohm's law $(I = E/R)$, is used for networks of electrical resistances. Resistance networks of any complexity can be analyzed by repeatedly applying the series and parallel resistance formulas given below.

When vessels with individual resistances $R_1, R_2, \ldots, R_n$ are connected in series, the overall resistance of the network is given by the following formula:

$$R_x = R_1 + R_2 + \ldots + R_n$$

Figure 7-2A shows an example of these vessels connected in series between some region where the pressure is P_i and another region with a lower pressure P_o, so that the total pressure difference across the network, ΔP, is equal to $P_i - P_o$. By the series resistance equation, the total resistance across the network (R_s) is equal to $R_1 + R_2 + R_3$. By the basic flow equation, the flow through the network $(\dot{Q})$ is equal to $\Delta P/R_s$. It should be intuitively obvious that $\dot{Q}$ is the flow (volume/time) through each of the elements in the series as indicated in Fig. 7-2B. [Fluid particles may move with different velocities (distance/time) in different elements in the network but the volume which passes through each element in a minute must be identical.]

As shown in Fig. 7-2C, a portion of the total pressure drop across the network occurs within each element of the series. The pressure drop across any element in the series can be calculated by applying the basic flow equation to that element, e.g., $\Delta P_1 = \dot{Q} R_1$. Note that the largest portion of the overall pressure

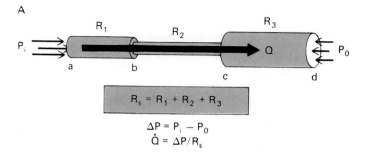

A

$$R_s = R_1 + R_2 + R_3$$

$$\Delta P = P_i - P_0$$
$$\dot{Q} = \Delta P / R_s$$

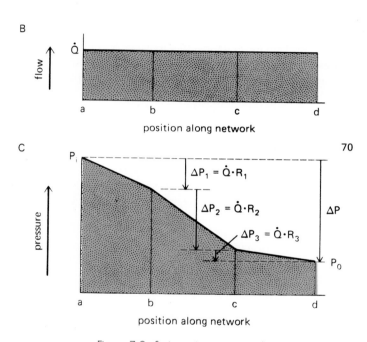

Figure 7-2 Series resistance network.

drop will occur across the element in the series with the largest resistance to flow (R_2 in Fig. 7-2).

As indicated in Fig. 7-3, when several tubes with individual resistances R_1, $R_2, \ldots, R_n$ are brought together to form a parallel network of vessels, one can calculate a single overall resistance for the parallel network R_p according to the following formula:

$$\frac{1}{R_p} = \frac{1}{R_1} + \frac{1}{R_2} + \ldots + \frac{1}{R_n}$$

The total flow through a parallel network is determined by $\Delta P/R_p$. As the preceding equation implies, the overall resistance of any parallel network will always be less than that of any of the elements in the network. (In the special case where the individual elements which form the network have identical resistances R_x, the overall resistance of the network is equal to the resistance of an individual element divided by the number of n of parallel elements in the network: $R_p = R_x/n$.) In general, the more parallel elements that occur in the network, the lower the overall resistance of the network. Thus, for example, a capillary bed which consists of many individual capillary vessels in parallel can have a very low overall resistance to flow even though the resistance of a single capillary is relatively high.

As indicated in Fig. 7-3, the basic flow equation may be applied to any single element in the network or to the network as a whole. For example, the flow through only the first element of the network ($\dot{Q}_1$) is given by $\dot{Q}_1 = \Delta P/R_1$, whereas the flow through the entire parallel network is given by $\dot{Q}_p = \Delta P/R_p$.

The series and parallel resistance equations may be utilized alternately to analyze resistance networks of great complexity. For example, any or all of the series resistances shown in Fig. 7-2 could actually represent the calculated overall resistance of many vessels arranged in parallel.

Blood Flow versus Blood Flow Velocity

Before proceeding, it is important to make the distinction between blood flow (volume/time) and blood flow velocity (distance/time) in the peripheral vascular system. Consider the analogy of a stream whose water moves with greater veloc-

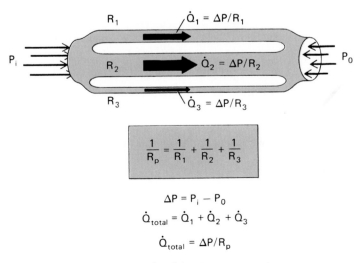

Figure 7-3   Parallel resistance network.

ity through a shallow rapids than it does through an adjacent deep pool. The volume of water passing through the pool in a day (volume/time = flow), however, must equal that passing through the rapids in the same day. In such a series arrangement, the flow is the same at all points along the channel but the flow velocity varies inversely with the local cross-sectional area. The situation is the same in the peripheral vasculature, where blood flows most rapidly in the region with the smallest total cross-sectional area (the aorta) and most slowly in the region with the largest total cross-sectional area (the capillary beds). Regardless of the differences in velocity, when the cardiac output (flow into the aorta) is 5 liters/min, the flow through the systemic capillaries (or arterioles, or venules) is also 5 liters/min. The changes in flow velocity that occur as blood passes through the peripheral vascular system are shown in the top trace of Fig. 7-4. These are a direct consequence of the variations in total cross-sectional area indicated in Fig. 7-1. The low capillary flow velocity maximizes the amount of time available for transcapillary exchange.

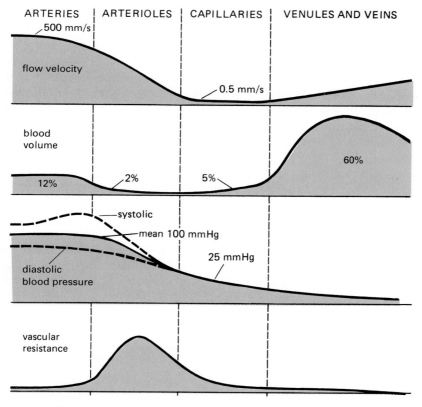

Figure 7-4 Flow velocities, blood volumes, blood pressures, and vascular resistances in the peripheral vasculature from aorta to right atrium.

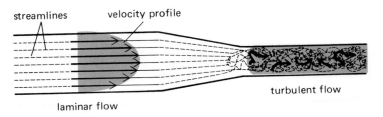

Figure 7-5   Laminar and turbulent flow patterns.

Laminar versus Turbulent Flow

Blood normally flows through all vessels in the cardiovascular system in an orderly streamlined manner called *laminar flow.* With laminar flow, there is a parabolic velocity profile across the tube as shown on the left side of Fig. 7-5. Velocity is fastest along the central axis of the tube and falls to zero at the wall. The concentric layers of fluid with different velocities slip smoothly over one another. Little mixing occurs between fluid layers so that individual particles move in straight streamlines parallel to the axis of the flow. Laminar flow is very efficient because little energy is wasted on anything but producing forward fluid motion.

Because blood is a viscous fluid, its movement through a vessel exerts a *shear stress* on the walls of the vessel. This is a force that wants to drag the inside surface (the endothelial cell layer) of the vessel along with the flow. With laminar flow, the shear stress on the wall of a vessel is proportional to the rate of flow through it.[1] The endothelial cells that line a vessel are able to sense (and thus respond to) changes in the rate of blood flow through the vessel by sensing changes in the shear stress on them. Shear stress may also be an important factor in certain pathological situations. For example, atherosclerotic plaques tend to form preferentially near branches off large arteries where, for complex hemodynamic reasons beyond the scope of this text, high shear stresses exist.

When blood is forced to move with high velocity through a narrow opening, the normal laminar flow pattern may break down into the *turbulent flow* pattern shown on the right side of Fig. 7-5.[2] With turbulent flow there is much internal mixing and friction. When the flow within a vessel is turbulent, the vessel's resistance to flow is significantly higher than that predicted from the

---

[1]   With pure laminar flow of a homogeneous fluid in a uniform smooth round tube, the shear stress (σ_s) on the wall is a function of fluid viscosity (η), flow (volume/time, Q), and the inside radius of the tube (r_i) as follows: $\sigma_s = 4\eta \dot{Q}/\pi r_i^3$.

[2]   Turbulence occurs when a parameter called the Reynolds number (R_e) exceeds a value of 2000. $R_e = 4\rho\dot{Q}/\pi\eta d_i$, where ρ = fluid density, Q = flow (volume-time), η = fluid viscosity, and d_i = inside diameter.

Poiseuille equation given in Chap. 1. Turbulent flow also generates sound, which can be heard with the aid of a stethoscope. For example, cardiac murmurs are manifestations of turbulent flow patterns generated by cardiac valve abnormalities. Detection of sounds (bruits) from peripheral arteries is abnormal and usually indicates significant reduction of the vessel's cross-sectional area.

Peripheral Blood Volumes

The second trace in Fig. 7-4 shows the approximate percentage of the total circulating blood volume that is contained in the different vascular regions of the systemic organs at any instant of time. (Approximately 20 percent of the total volume is contained in the pulmonary system and the heart chambers and is not accounted for in this figure.) Note that most of the circulating blood is contained within the veins of the systemic organs. This diffuse but large blood reservoir is often referred to as the *peripheral venous pool.* A second but smaller reservoir of venous blood, called the *central venous pool,* is contained in the great veins of the thorax and the right atrium. When peripheral veins constrict, blood is displaced from the peripheral venous pool and enters the central pool. An increase in the central venous volume, and thus pressure, enhances cardiac filling, which in turn augments stroke volume according to the Frank-Starling law of the heart. This is an extremely important mechanism of cardiovascular regulation and will be discussed in greater detail in Chap. 9.

Peripheral Blood Pressures

Blood pressure decreases in the consecutive segments with the pattern shown in the third trace of Fig. 7-4. Recall from Fig. 4-1 that aortic pressure fluctuates between a systolic and diastolic value with each heartbeat, and the same is true throughout the arterial system. (For complex hemodynamic reasons, the difference between systolic and diastolic pressure actually increases with the distance from the heart in the large arteries.[3]) The average pressure in the root of the aorta, however, is about 100 mmHg, and this *mean arterial pressure* falls by only a small amount within the arterial system.

A large pressure drop occurs in the arterioles, where in addition the pulsatile nature of the pressure nearly disappears. The mean capillary pressure is approximately 25 mmHg. Pressure continues to decrease in the

---

[3] A rigorous analysis of the dynamics of pulsatile fluid flow in tapered, branching, elastic tubes is required to explain such behavior. Pressure does not increase simultaneously throughout the arterial system with the onset of cardiac ejection. Rather, the pressure increase begins at the root of the aorta and travels outward from there. When this rapidly moving pressure wave encounters obstacles such as vessel bifurcations, reflected waves are generated which travel back toward the heart. These reflected waves can summate with and reinforce the oncoming wave in a manner somewhat analogous to the progressive cresting of surface waves as they impinge on a beach.

venules and veins as blood returns to the right heart. The central venous
pressure (which is the filling pressure for the right heart) is normally very
close to 0 mmHg.

Peripheral Vascular Resistances

The bottom trace in Fig. 7-4 indicates the relative resistance to flow that exists in
each of the consecutive vascular regions. Recall from Chap. 1 that resistance,
pressure difference, and flow are related by the basic flow equation $\dot{Q} = \Delta P/R$.
Since the flow $(\dot{Q})$ must be the same through each of the consecutive regions indicated in Fig. 7-4, the pressure drop which occurs across each of these regions
is a direct reflection of the resistance to flow within that region (see Fig. 7-2).
Thus, the large pressure drop occurring as blood moves through arterioles indicates that arterioles present a large resistance to flow. The mean pressure drops
little in arteries because they have little resistance to flow. Similarly, the modest
pressure drop which exists across capillaries is a reflection of the fact that the
capillary bed has a modest resistance to flow when compared to that of the arteriolar bed. (Recall from Fig. 7-3 that the capillary bed can have a low resistance
to flow because it is a parallel network of a very large number of individual capillaries.)

   Blood flow through many individual organs can vary over a 10-fold or
greater range. Since mean arterial pressure is a relatively stable cardiovascular variable, large changes in an organ's blood flow must result from changes
in its overall vascular resistance to blood flow. The consecutive vascular segments are arranged in series within an organ, and the overall vascular resistance of the organ must equal the sum of the resistances of its consecutive
vascular segments:

$$R_{organ} = R_{arteries} + R_{arterioles} + R_{capillaries} + R_{venules} + R_{veins}$$

Since arterioles have such a large vascular resistance in comparison to the other
vascular segments, the overall vascular resistance of any organ is determined to a
very large extent by the resistance of its arterioles. Arteriolar resistance is, of
course, strongly influenced by arteriolar radius (R is proportional to $1/r^4$). Thus
the blood flow through an organ is primarily regulated by adjustments in the internal diameter of arterioles caused by contraction or relaxation of the muscular
arteriolar walls.

   When the arterioles of an organ change diameter, not only does the flow
to the organ change but the manner in which the pressures drop within the organ is also modified. The effects of arteriolar dilation and constriction on the
pressure profile within a vascular bed are illustrated in Fig. 7-6. Arteriolar
constriction causes a greater pressure drop across the arterioles and this tends
to increase the arterial pressure while it decreases the pressure in capillaries

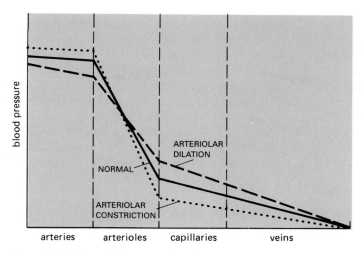

Figure 7-6   Effect of changes in arteriolar resistance on vascular pressures.

and veins. (The arterioles function somewhat like a dam; closing a dam's gates decreases the flow while increasing the level of the reservoir behind it and decreasing the level of its outflow stream.) Conversely, increased organ blood flow caused by arteriolar dilation is accompanied by decreased arterial pressure and increased capillary pressure. Because of the changes in capillary hydrostatic pressure, arteriolar constriction tends to cause transcapillary fluid reabsorption whereas arteriolar dilation tends to promote transcapillary fluid filtration.

Total Peripheral Resistance

The overall resistance to flow through the entire systemic circulation is called the *total peripheral resistance.* Since the systemic organs are generally arranged in parallel (Fig. 1-2), the vascular resistance of each organ contributes to the total peripheral resistance according to the following parallel resistance equation:

$$\frac{1}{R_p} = \frac{1}{R_1} + \frac{1}{R_2} + \ldots + \frac{1}{R_n}$$

As will be discussed later in this chapter, the total peripheral resistance is an important determinant of arterial blood pressure.

Elastic Properties of Vessels

As indicated earlier, arteries and veins contribute only a small portion to the overall resistance to flow through a vascular bed. Therefore, we are usually not concerned with the minor influences which changes in their diameters have on the blood flow through systemic organs. The elastic behavior of arteries and veins is, however, very important to overall cardiovascular function because they can act as reservoirs and substantial amounts of blood can be stored in them.

The elastic properties of vessels or vascular regions are often characterized by a parameter called *compliance (C),* which describes how much their volume changes (ΔV) in response to a given change in transmural pressure (ΔP):

$$C = \frac{\Delta V}{\Delta P}$$

Transmural pressure is the difference between the internal and external pressures on the vessel wall.

The elastic properties of veins are important to their blood reservoir function. As indicated by the volume-pressure curves in Fig. 7-7, veins are much more compliant than arteries. Because veins are so compliant, even small changes in peripheral venous pressure can cause a significant amount of the circulating blood volume to shift into or out of the peripheral venous pool. Standing upright, for example, increases venous pressure in the lower extremities and promotes blood accumulation (pooling) in these vessels as might be represented by a shift from point A to point B in Fig. 7-7. Fortunately this process can be counteracted by active venous constriction. The dashed line in Fig. 7-7 shows

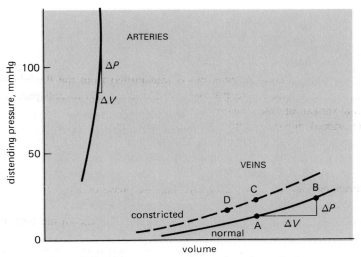

Figure 7-7   Volume-pressure curves of arteries and veins.

the venous volume-pressure relationship that exists when veins are constricted by activation of venous smooth muscle. In constricted veins, volume may be normal (point C) or even below normal (point D) despite higher than normal venous pressure. Peripheral venous constriction per se tends to increase peripheral venous pressure and shift blood out of the peripheral venous reservoir.

The elastic properties of arteries allow them to act as a reservoir on a beat-to-beat basis. Arteries play an important role in converting the pulsatile flow output of the heart into a steady flow through the vascular beds of systemic organs. In this regard arteries are said to serve a *windkessel* (German for air chamber) *function.* During the early rapid phase of cardiac ejection, the arterial volume increases because blood is entering the aorta more rapidly than it is passing into systemic arterioles. Thus, part of the work the heart does in ejecting blood goes to stretching the elastic walls of arteries. Toward the end of systole and throughout diastole, arterial volume decreases because the flow out of arteries exceeds flow into the aorta. Previously stretched arterial walls recoil to shorter lengths, and in the process give up their stored potential energy. This reconverted energy is what actually does the work of propelling blood through the peripheral vascular beds during diastole. If the arteries were rigid tubes which could not store energy by expanding elastically, arterial pressure would fall immediately to zero with the termination of each cardiac ejection.

MEASUREMENT OF ARTERIAL PRESSURE

Recall that the systemic arterial pressure fluctuates with each heart cycle between a diastolic value (P_D) and a higher systolic value (P_S). Obtaining estimates of an individual's systolic and diastolic pressures is one of the most routine diagnostic techniques available to the physician. The basic principles of the *auscultation* technique used to measure blood pressure are described here with the aid of Fig. 7-8.

An inflatable cuff is wrapped around the upper arm, and a device, such as a mercury manometer, is attached to monitor the pressure within the cuff. The cuff is initially inflated with air to a pressure ($\approx$175 to 200 mmHg) that is well above normal systolic values. This pressure is transmitted from the flexible cuff into the upper arm tissues, where it causes all blood vessels to collapse. No blood flows into (or out of) the forearm as long as the cuff pressure is higher than the systolic arterial pressure. After the initial inflation, air is allowed to gradually "bleed" from the cuff so that the pressure within it falls slowly and steadily through the range of arterial pressure fluctuations. The moment the cuff pressure falls below the peak systolic arterial pressure, some blood is able to pass through the arteries beneath the cuff during the systolic phase of the cycle. This flow is intermittent and occurs only over a brief period of each heart cycle. Moreover, because it occurs through partially collapsed vessels beneath the cuff, the flow is turbulent rather than laminar. The intermittent periods of flow beneath the cuff produce tapping sounds, which can be detected with a stethoscope placed over the radial artery at the elbow. As indicated in Fig. 7-8, sounds of varying

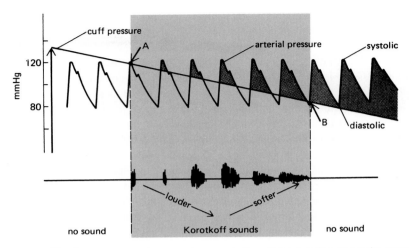

Figure 7-8 Blood pressure measurement by auscultation. Point A indicates systolic pressure and point B indicates diastolic pressure.

character, known collectively as *Korotkoff sounds,* are heard whenever the cuff pressure is between the systolic and diastolic aortic pressures.

Since there is no blood flow and thus no sound when cuff pressure is higher than systolic arterial pressure, *the highest cuff pressure at which tapping sounds are heard is taken as the systolic arterial pressure.* When the cuff pressure falls below the diastolic pressure, blood flows through the vessels beneath the cuff without periodic interruption and again no sound is detected over the radial artery. *The cuff pressure at which the sounds become muffled or disappear is taken as the diastolic arterial pressure.* The Korotkoff sounds are more distinct when the cuff pressure is near the systolic arterial pressure than when it is near the diastolic pressure. Thus consistency in determining diastolic pressure by auscultation requires concentration and experience.

DETERMINANTS OF ARTERIAL PRESSURE

Mean Arterial Pressure

Mean arterial pressure is a critically important cardiovascular variable because it is the average effective pressure that drives blood through the systemic organs. One of the most fundamental equations of cardiovascular physiology is that which indicates how mean arterial pressure $(\overline{P}_A)$ is related to cardiac output (CO) and total peripheral resistance (TPR):

$$\overline{P}_A = \text{CO} \times \text{TPR}$$

As illustrated in Fig. 7-9A, this equation is simply a rearrangement of the basic flow equation $(\dot{Q} = \Delta P/R)$ applied to the entire systemic circulation with the single assumption that central venous pressure is approximately zero so that $\Delta P = \bar{P}_A$. Note that mean arterial pressure is influenced both by the heart (via cardiac output) and by the peripheral vasculature (via total peripheral resistance). *All changes in mean arterial pressure result from changes in either cardiac output or total peripheral resistance.*

Fig. 7-9A shows how the normal mean arterial pressure at rest of 100 mmHg is a direct consequence of the facts that normal resting cardiac output is 5 liters/min and normal resting total peripheral resistance is 20 mmHg/liters/min. A decrease in TPR without a change in CO will necessarily result in a decrease in $\bar{P}_a$ as illustrated in Fig. 7-9B. Fig. 7-9C shows how a normal arterial pressure of 100 mmHg can be maintained in the face of decreased TPR by a compensatory increase in CO.

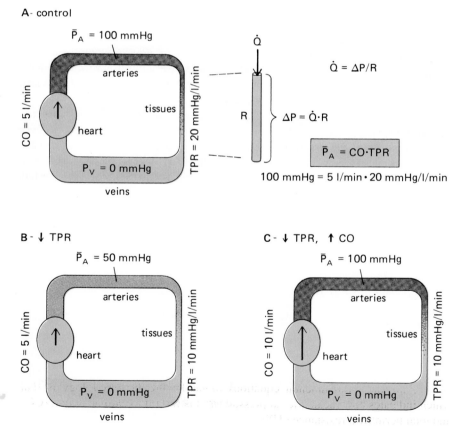

Figure 7-9 Determination of mean arterial pressure $(\bar{P}_A)$ by cardiac output (CO) and total peripheral resistance (TPR).

Calculating the true value of mean arterial pressure requires mathematically averaging the arterial pressure waveform over one or more complete heart cycles. Most often, however, we know from auscultation only the systolic and diastolic pressures, yet wish to make some estimate of the mean arterial pressure. Mean arterial pressure necessarily falls between the systolic and diastolic pressures. A useful rule of thumb is that mean arterial pressure $(\overline{P}_A)$ is approximately equal to diastolic pressure $(\overline{P}_O)$ plus one-third of the difference between systolic and diastolic pressure $(P_S - P_D)$:

$$\overline{P}_A \simeq P_D + \frac{1}{3}(P_S - P_D)$$

Arterial Pulse Pressure

The *arterial pulse pressure* (P_p) is defined simply as systolic pressure minus diastolic pressure:

$$P_p = P_S - P_D$$

To be able to use pulse pressure to deduce something about how the cardiovascular system is operating we must do more than just define it. We must understand what determines pulse pressure; i.e., what causes it to be what it is and what can cause it to change? In a previous section of this chapter we discussed briefly how, as a consequence of the compliance of the arterial vessels, arterial pressure increases as arterial blood volume is expanded during cardiac ejection. The magnitude of the pressure increase (ΔP) caused by an increase in arterial volume depends on how large the volume change (ΔV) is and on how compliant (C_A) the arterial space is: $\Delta P = \Delta V/C_A$. If, for the moment, we neglect the fact that some blood leaves the arterial space *during* cardiac ejection, then the increase in arterial volume during each heartbeat is equal to the stroke volume (SV). Thus pulse pressure is, to a first approximation, equal to stroke volume divided by arterial compliance:

$$P_P \simeq \frac{SV}{C_A}$$

Pulse pressure tends to increase with age in adults because of a decrease in arterial compliance ("hardening of the arteries"). Arterial volume-pressure curves for a 20-year-old and a 70-year-old are shown in Fig. 7-10. The decrease in arterial compliance with age is indicated by the steeper curve for the 70-year-old (more ΔP for a given ΔV) than for the 20-year-old. Thus, a 70-year-old will necessarily have a larger pulse pressure for a given stroke volume than a 20-year-old. As indicated in Fig. 7-10, the decrease in arterial compliance is sufficient to cause increased pulse pressure even though stroke volume tends to decrease with age. (Figure 7-10 also illustrates the fact that arterial blood volume

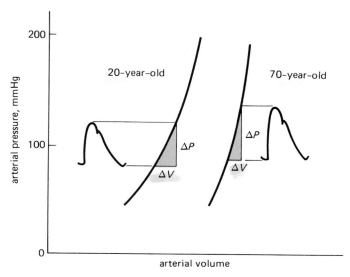

Figure 7-10   Effect of age on the arterial volume-pressure relationship.

and mean arterial pressure tend to increase with age. The increase in mean arterial pressure is *not* caused by the decreased arterial compliance, however, since compliance changes do not directly influence cardiac output or TPR which are the *sole determinants* of $\bar{P}_A$. Mean arterial pressure tends to increase with age because of an age-dependent increase in TPR.)

Arterial compliance also decreases with increasing mean arterial pressure as evidenced by the curvature of the volume-pressure relationships shown in Fig. 7-10. Otherwise, arterial compliance is a relatively stable parameter. Thus most acute changes in arterial pulse pressure are the result of changes in stroke volume.

The preceding equation for pulse pressure is a much simplified description of some very complex hemodynamic processes. It correctly identifies stroke volume and arterial compliance as the major determinants of arterial pulse pressure but is based on the assumption that no blood leaves the aorta during systolic ejection. Obviously this is not strictly correct. Furthermore, close examination of Fig. 4-1 will reveal that peak systolic pressure is reached even before cardiac ejection is complete. It is therefore not surprising that several factors other than arterial compliance and stroke volume have minor influences on pulse pressure. For example, faster cardiac ejection caused by increased myocardial contractility tends to increase pulse pressure somewhat even if stroke volume remains constant. Changes in total peripheral resistance, however, have *little or no effect on pulse pressure,* since a change in TPR causes parallel changes in both systolic and diastolic pressure.

A common misconception in cardiovascular physiology is that the systolic pressure alone or the diastolic pressure alone indicates the status of a specific cardiovascular variable. For example, high diastolic pressure is often taken to indicate high total peripheral resistance. This is not necessarily so since high diastolic pressure can exist with normal (or even reduced) TPR if heart rate and cardiac output are high. Both systolic pressure and diastolic pressure are influenced by heart rate, stroke volume, TPR, and C_A.[4] The student should not attempt to interpret systolic and diastolic pressure values independently. Interpretation is much more straightforward when the focus is on mean arterial pressure ($\bar{P}_A$ = CO × TPR) and arterial pulse pressure ($P_p \simeq SV/C_A$). (See study question 34.)

Study Questions: 24 to 34

---

[4]   The equations presented in this and preceding chapters can be solved simultaneously to show that

$$P_S \simeq SV \times HR \times TPR + \frac{2}{3}\frac{SV}{C_A}$$

$$P_D \simeq SV \times HR \times TPR - \frac{1}{3}\frac{SV}{C_A}$$

8

VASCULAR CONTROL

OBJECTIVES

The student understands the general mechanisms involved in local vascular control:

1 Identifies the major ways in which smooth muscle differs anatomically and functionally from striated muscle.
2 Lists the steps leading to cross-bridge cycling in smooth muscle.
3 Lists the major ion channels involved in the regulation of membrane potential in smooth muscle.
4 Describes the processes of electromechanical and pharmacomechanical coupling in smooth muscle.
5 Defines basal tone.
6 Lists several substances potentially involved in local metabolic control.
7 States the local metabolic vasodilator hypothesis.
8 Describes how vascular tone is influenced by prostaglandins, histamine, and bradykinin.
9 Describes the myogenic response of blood vessels.
10 Defines active and reactive hyperemia and indicates a possible mechanism for each.
11 Defines autoregulation of blood flow and briefly describes the metabolic, myogenic, and tissue pressure theories of autoregulation.
12 Defines neurogenic tone and describes how sympathetic (and parasympathetic) neural influences can alter it.
13 Describes how vascular tone is influenced by circulating catecholamines, vasopressin, and angiotensin II.
14 Lists the major influences on venous diameters.
15 Describes in general how control of flow differs between organs with strong local metabolic control of arteriolar tone and organs with strong neurogenic control of arteriolar tone.

The student knows the dominant mechanisms of flow and blood volume control in the major body organs:

16 States the relative importance of local metabolic and neural control of coronary blood flow.
17 Defines systolic compression and indicates its relative importance to blood flow in the endocardial and epicardial regions of the right and left ventricular walls.
18 Describes the major mechanisms of flow and blood volume control in each of the following specific systemic organs: skeletal muscle, brain, splanchnic organs, skin, and kidney.
19 States why mean pulmonary arterial pressure is lower than mean systemic arterial pressure.
20 Describes how pulmonary vascular control differs from that in systemic organs.
21 Identifies the pathway of blood flow through the fetal heart and describes the changes that occur at birth.

VASCULAR SMOOTH MUSCLE

Because the body's metabolic needs are continually changing, the cardiovascular system must continually make adjustments in the diameter of its blood vessels. The purposes of these vascular changes are to (1) control the rate of blood flow through particular tissues (the job of arterioles) and (2) regulate the distribution of blood volume and cardiac filling (the job of veins). These diameter adjustments are made by regulating the contractile activity of vascular smooth muscle cells which are present in the walls of all vessels except capillaries. The task of vascular smooth muscle is unique because to maintain a certain vessel diameter in the face of the continual distending pressure of the blood within it, vascular smooth muscle must be able to sustain active tension for prolonged periods.

There are many functional characteristics that distinguish smooth muscle from either skeletal or cardiac muscle. For example, when compared to these other muscle types, smooth muscle cells:

1 contract and relax much more slowly.
2 develop active tension over a greater range of muscle lengths.
3 can change their contractile activity as the result of action potentials *or* changes in resting membrane potential.
4 may change their contractile activity in the absence of changes in membrane potential.
5 maintain tension for prolonged periods at low energy cost.
6 can be activated by stretch.

Contractile Machinery

Vascular smooth muscle cells are small (about 5 μm $\times$ 50 μm) spindle-shaped cells usually arranged circumferentially in blood vessel walls. In many vessels, adjacent smooth muscle cells are electrically connected by gap junctions similar to those found in the myocardium.

Just as in other muscle types, smooth muscle force development and shortening are the result of cross-bridge interaction between thick and thin contractile filaments composed of myosin and actin, respectively. In smooth muscle, however, these filaments are not arranged in regular, repeating sarcomere units. As a consequence, "smooth" muscle cells lack the microscopically visible striations characteristic of skeletal and cardiac muscle cells. The actin filaments in smooth muscle are much longer than those in striated muscle. Many of these actin filaments attach to the inner surface of the cell at structures called *dense bands*. In the interior of the cell, actin filaments are connected together in small bundles by transverse structures called *dense bodies*. Myosin filaments are interspersed between the smooth muscle actin filaments but in a more haphazard fashion than the regular interleaving pattern of striated muscle. In striated muscle, the contractile filaments are invariably aligned with the long axis of the cell whereas in smooth muscle many contractile filaments travel obliquely or even transversely to the long axis of the cell. Despite the absence of organized sarcomeres, changes in smooth muscle length affect its ability to actively develop tension. Perhaps because of the long actin filaments and the lack of sarcomere arrangement, smooth muscle can develop tension over a greater range of length than either skeletal or cardiac muscle.

As in striated muscle, the strength of the cross-bridge interaction between thick and thin filaments in smooth muscle is controlled primarily by changes in the intracellular free Ca^{2+} level, which range from about 10^{-7} M in relaxed muscle to 10^{-6} M during maximal contraction. However, the sequence of steps linking an increased free Ca^{2+} level to contractile filament interaction is different in smooth muscle than in striated muscle. In smooth muscle:

1 Ca^{2+} first forms a complex with the calcium binding protein *calmodulin.*
2 The Ca^{2+}-calmodulin complex then activates a phosphorylating enzyme called *myosin light chain kinase.*
3 This enzyme causes phosphorylation by adenosine triphosphate (ATP) of the light chain protein that is a portion of the cross-bridge head of myosin.
4 Myosin light chain phosphorylation enables cross-bridge formation and cycling during which energy from ATP is utilized for tension development and shortening.

Smooth muscle is also unique in that once tension is developed, it can be maintained at very low energy costs, i.e., without the need to continually split ATP in cross-bridge cycling. The mechanisms responsible are still somewhat unclear but presumably involve very slowly or even noncycling cross-bridges. This is often referred to as the *latch state* and may involve light chain dephosphorylation of attached cross-bridges. Also by mechanisms that are yet incompletely understood, it is apparent that vascular smooth muscle contractile activity is regulated not only by changes in intracellular free Ca^{2+} levels but also by changes in the *Ca^{2+} sensitivity* of the contractile machinery. Thus the contractile state of vascular smooth muscle may sometimes change in the absence of changes in intracellular free Ca^{2+} levels.

Membrane Potentials

Smooth muscle cells have resting membrane potentials ranging from -40 to -65 mV and thus are generally lower than those in striated muscle. As in all cells, the resting membrane potential of smooth muscle is determined largely by the cell permeability to potassium. Several types of K^+ channels have been identified in smooth muscle. The one predominantly responsible for determining the resting membrane potential is termed an *inward rectifying* type K^+ channel. (*Inward rectifying* signifies that K^+ ions move into cells through this channel more easily than they move out through it.) There is also an *ATP-dependent* K^+ channel that is closed when cellular ATP levels are normal but opens if ATP levels fall. This channel may be important in matching organ blood flow to the metabolic state of the tissue.

Smooth muscle cells regularly have action potentials only in certain vessels. When they do occur, smooth muscle action potentials are initiated primarily by inward Ca^{2+} current and are developed slowly like the "slow type" cardiac action potentials (see Fig. 3-3). As in the heart, this inward (depolarizing) Ca^{2+} current flows through a *voltage-operated calcium channel* (VOC); this type of channel is one of several types of calcium channels present in smooth muscle. The repolarization phase of the action potential occurs primarily by an outward flux of potassium ions through both *delayed rectifying* K^+ channels and *calcium-activated* K^+ channels.

Many types of ion channels in addition to those mentioned have been identified in vascular smooth muscle, but in most cases their exact role in cardiovascular function remains obscure. For example, there appear to be nonselective, stretch-sensitive cation channels which may be involved in the response of smooth muscle to stretch. The reader should note, however, that many of the important ion channels in vascular smooth muscle are also important in heart muscle (see Table 3-1).

Electromechanical versus Pharmacomechanical Coupling

In smooth muscle, changes in intracellular free Ca^{2+} levels can occur both with and without changes in membrane potential. The processes involved are called *electromechanical coupling* and *pharmacomechanical coupling,* respectively, and are illustrated in Fig. 8-1.

Electromechanical coupling, shown in the left half of Fig. 8-1, occurs because the smooth muscle surface membrane contains voltage-operated channels for calcium (the same VOCs that are involved in action potential generation). Membrane depolarization increases the open-state probability of these channels and thus leads to smooth muscle cell contraction and vessel constriction. Conversely, membrane hyperpolarization leads to smooth muscle relaxation and ves-

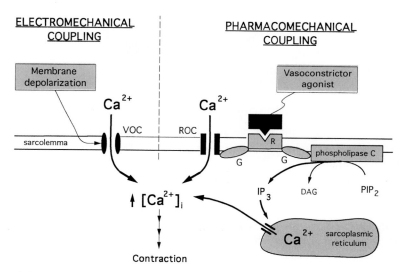

Figure 8-1 General mechanisms for activation of vascular smooth muscle. VOC, voltage-operated Ca^{2+} channel; ROC, receptor-operated Ca^{2+} channel; R, agonist specific receptor; G, GTP-binding protein; PIP_2, phosphatidyl inositol biphosphate; IP_3, inositol triphosphate; DAG, diacylglycerol.

sel dilation. Since the VOCs for Ca^{2+} are partially activated by the low resting membrane potential of vascular smooth muscle, changes in resting potential can alter the resting calcium influx rate and therefore the basal contractile state.

With pharmacomechanical coupling, chemical agents (e.g., released neurotransmitters) can induce smooth muscle contraction without the need for a change in membrane potential. As illustrated in the right side of Fig. 8-1, the combination of a vasoconstrictor agonist (such as norepinephrine) with a specific membrane-bound receptor (such as an α-adrenergic receptor) initiates events that cause intracellular free Ca^{2+} levels to increase for two reasons. One, the activated receptor may open surface membrane *receptor-operated channels* (ROCs) for Ca^{2+}, which allows Ca^{2+} influx from the extracellular fluid. Two, the activated receptor may induce the formation of an intracellular "second messenger," inositol trisphosphate (IP_3), which opens specific channels that release Ca^{2+} from the intracellular sarcoplasmic reticulum stores. In both processes, the activated receptor first stimulates specific guanosine triphosphate binding proteins (GTP-binding proteins or *"G proteins"*).

The reader should *not* conclude from Fig. 8-1 that all vasoactive chemical agents (chemical agents that cause vascular effects) produce their actions on smooth muscle without changing membrane potential. In fact, most vasoactive chemical agents do cause changes in membrane potential because their receptors can be linked, by G proteins or other means, to ion channels of many kinds.

Not shown in Fig. 8-1 are the processes that remove Ca^{2+} from the cytoplasm of vascular smooth muscle although they are important as well in determining the free cytosolic Ca^{2+} levels. As in cardiac cells (see Fig. 3-7), smooth muscle cells actively pump calcium into the sarcoplasmic reticulum and outward across the sarcolemma. Calcium is also countertransported out of the cell in exchange for sodium.

Mechanisms for Relaxation

Hyperpolarization of the cell membrane is one mechanism for causing smooth muscle relaxation and vessel dilation. In addition, however, there are at least two general mechanisms by which certain chemical vasodilator agents can cause smooth muscle relaxation by pharmacomechanical means. In Fig. 8-1, the receptor for a chemical vasoconstrictor agent was linked by a specific G protein to phospholipase C. In an analogous manner, other specific receptors may be linked by other specific G proteins to other enzymes which produce second messengers other than IP_3. An important example is the β_2-adrenergic receptor of smooth muscle which is linked by a particular G protein (G_s) to adenylate cyclase. Adenylate cyclase catalyses the conversion of ATP to cyclic adenosine monophosphate (cAMP). In smooth muscle, cAMP is a second messenger which tends to reduce intracellular free Ca^{2+} concentration by somehow stimulating the rate at which calcium is pumped out of the cell and into the sarcoplasmic reticulum.

In addition to cAMP, cyclic guanosine monophosphate (cGMP) is an important second messenger that causes vascular smooth muscle relaxation by mechanisms that are not yet clear. Formed from GTP by the action of guanylate cyclase, cGMP is an intracellular enzyme that can be activated by an important vasodilator substance, nitric oxide (NO), which is produced by endothelial cells. Nitroglycerine is a clinically important vasodilator drug that acts through a similar mechanism.

Vascular Tone

Vascular tone is a term commonly used to characterize the general contractile state of a vessel or a vascular region. For our purposes, the "vascular tone" of a region can be taken as an indication of the "level of activation" of the individual smooth muscle cells in that region. Actually, this association is a statistical one because rarely do all the cells in a vessel or all the vessels in a vascular region act in precise unison.

CONTROL OF ARTERIOLAR ZONE

As described in Chap. 7, the blood flow through any organ is determined largely by its vascular resistance, which is dependent primarily on the diameter of its arterioles. Consequently, an organ's flow is controlled by factors that influence the arteriolar smooth muscle tone.

Arterioles remain in a state of partial constriction even when all external influences on them are removed; hence they are said to have a degree of *basal tone*. Our understanding of the mechanism is vague, but basal arteriolar tone may be a reflection of the fact that smooth muscle cells inherently and actively resist being stretched as they continually are in pressurized arterioles. In any case, this basal tone establishes a baseline of partial arteriolar constriction from which the external influences on arterioles exert their dilating or constricting effects. These influences can be separated into three categories: local influences, neural influences, and hormonal influences.

Local Influences on Arterioles

Local Metabolic Influences   The arterioles that control flow through a given organ lie within the organ tissue itself. Thus, arterioles and the smooth muscle in their walls are exposed to the chemical composition of the interstitial fluid of the organ they serve. The interstitial concentrations of many substances reflect the balance between the metabolic activity of the tissue and its blood supply. Interstitial oxygen levels, for example, fall whenever the tissue cells are utilizing oxygen faster than it is being supplied to the tissue by blood flow. Conversely, interstitial oxygen levels rise whenever excess oxygen is being delivered to a tissue from the blood. In nearly all vascular beds, exposure to low oxygen reduces arteriolar tone and causes vasodilation, whereas high oxygen levels cause arteriolar vasoconstriction.[1] Thus a local feedback mechanism exists that automatically operates on arterioles to regulate a tissue's blood flow in accordance with its metabolic needs. Whenever blood flow and oxygen delivery fall below a tissue's oxygen demands, the oxygen levels around arterioles fall, the arterioles dilate, and the blood flow through the organ appropriately increases.

The ATP-sensitive K^+ channels of smooth muscle cells may represent one mechanism by which changes in tissues metabolic needs lead to changes in arteriolar tone. Consider, for example, the following sequence of events: (1) any tissue underperfusion would cause decreased ATP levels in the vascular smooth muscle cell; (2) low ATP levels open ATP-dependent K^+ channels; (3) opening any K^+ channel causes hyperpolarization; (4) hyperpolarization closes voltage-dependent Ca^{2+} channels; (5) cytosolic free Ca^{2+} levels fall; (6) the level of smooth muscle cell activation decreases; (7) vessels dilate; and (8) blood flow increases to more adequately meet the metabolic needs of the tissue.

Many substances in addition to oxygen are present within tissues and can affect the tone of vascular smooth muscle. When the metabolic rate of skeletal muscle is increased by exercise, for example, not only do tissue levels of O_2 decrease, but those of CO_2, H^+, and K^+ increase. Muscle tissue osmolarity also increases during exercise. All of these chemical alterations cause arteriolar dilation. In addition, with increased metabolic activity or oxygen deprivation, cells

---

[1]   An important exception to this rule occurs in the pulmonary circulation and will be discussed later in this chapter.

in many tissues may release *adenosine,* which is an extremely potent vasodilator agent.

At present we do not know which of these (or possibly other) metabolically related chemical alterations within tissues are most important in the local metabolic control of blood flow. It appears likely that arteriolar tone depends on the combined action of many factors. In addition, any given factor may have different degrees of importance in the local metabolic control of flow in different organs.

For conceptual purposes, our understanding of local metabolic control can be summarized as shown in Fig. 8-2. Vasodilator factors enter the interstitial space from the tissue cells at a rate proportional to tissue metabolism. These vasodilator factors are removed from the tissue at a rate proportional to blood flow. Whenever tissue metabolism is proceeding at a rate for which the blood flow is inadequate, the interstitial vasodilator factor concentrations automatically build up and cause the arterioles to dilate. This, of course, causes blood flow to increase. The process continues until blood flow has risen sufficiently to appropriately match the tissue metabolic rate and prevent further accumulation of vasodilator factors. The same system also operates to reduce blood flow when it is higher than required by the tissue's metabolic activity, because this situation causes a reduction in the interstitial concentrations of metabolic vasodilator factors.

Local Influences from Endothelial Cells   Endothelial cells cover the entire inner surface of the cardiovascular system. A large number of studies have shown that blood vessels respond very differently to certain vascular influences when their endothelial lining is missing. Acetylcholine, for example, causes vasodilation of intact vessels but causes vasoconstriction of vessels stripped of their endothelial lining. This and other similar results have led to the realization that endothelial cells respond to various stimuli by producing a local factor

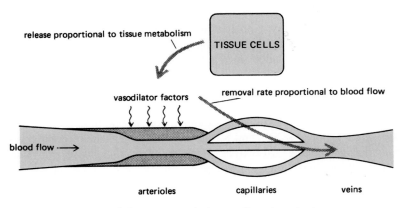

Figure 8-2   Local metabolic vasodilator hypothesis.

that can decrease the tone of the overlying smooth muscle layers. Originally called EDRF (endothelial derived relaxing factor), this substance has now been identified as NO. It is produced within endothelial cells from the amino acid, L-arginine, by the action of an enzyme, NO synthase. Nitric oxide synthase is activated by a rise in the intracellular level of the Ca^{2+}. Nitric oxide is a small lipid-soluble molecule that, once formed, easily diffuses into adjacent smooth muscle cells where it is thought to cause relaxation by stimulating cGMP production.

Acetylcholine and several other agents (including bradykinin, vasoactive intestinal peptide, and substance P) stimulate endothelial cell NO production because their receptors on endothelial cells are linked to receptor-operated Ca^{2+} channels. Probably more importantly from a physiological standpoint, flow-related shear stresses on endothelial cells stimulates their NO production presumably because stretch-sensitive channels for Ca^{2+} are activated. Such flow-related endothelial cell NO production probably explains why, for example, exercise and increased blood flow through muscles of the lower leg can cause dilation of the blood-supplying femoral artery at points far upstream of the exercising muscle itself.

Agents that block NO production by inhibiting NO synthase cause significant increases in the vascular resistances of most resting organs. For this reason, it is believed that endothelial cells are normally always producing some NO that is importantly involved, along with other factors, in determining the normal net resting tone of arterioles throughout the body.

By mechanisms that are presently not well understood, endothelial cells also produce another relaxing agent (presently called "endothelial-derived hyperpolarizing factor") and several constrictor factors including *endothelin*, a very potent constrictor peptide. The physiological roles of these agents have not yet been established.

Other Local Chemical Influences   In addition to the local metabolic influences on vascular tone, many specific chemical substances have been identified which have vascular effects and therefore could be important in local vascular regulation in certain instances. In most cases, however, definite information about the relative importance of these substances in cardiovascular regulation is lacking.

Prostaglandins are a group of several chemically related products of the cyclooxygenase pathway of arachadonic acid metabolism. Certain prostaglandins are potent vasodilators while others are potent vasoconstrictors. Despite the vasoactive potency of the prostaglandins and the fact that most tissues (including endothelial cells and vascular smooth muscle cells) are capable of synthesizing prostaglandins, it has not been demonstrated convincingly that prostaglandins play a crucial role in *normal* vascular control. It is clear however that vasodilator prostaglandins are involved in inflammatory responses. Consequently, inhibitors of prostaglandin synthesis, such as aspirin, are effective anti-inflammatory drugs. Prostaglandins produced by platelets and endothelial cells are important in the hemostatic (flow stopping, antibleeding) vasoconstrictor and platelet-aggregating responses to vascular injury. Hence, aspirin is often prescribed to reduce the tendency for blood clotting—especially in patients with potential coronary flow limitations. Arachadonic acid metabolites produced via the lipoxygenase system (e.g., *leukotrienes*) also have vasoactive properties and may influence blood flow under certain conditions.

Histamine is synthesized and stored in high concentrations in secretory granules of tissue mast cells and circulating basophils. When released, histamine produces arteriolar vasodilation and increases vascular permeability, which leads to edema formation and local tissue swelling. Histamine increases vascular permeability by causing separations in the junctions between the endothelial cells which line the vascular system. Histamine release is classically associated with *antigen-antibody reactions* in various allergic and immune responses. Many drugs and physical or chemical insults which damage tissue also cause histamine release. Histamine can stimulate sensory nerve endings to cause itching and pain sensations. While clearly important in many pathological situations, it seems unlikely that histamine participates in normal cardiovascular regulation.

Bradykinin and *kallidin* are polypeptides which have about 10 times the vasodilator potency of histamine on a molar basis. These kinins also act to increase capillary permeability by opening the junctions between endothelial cells. They are formed from certain plasma globulin substrates by the action of an enzyme, *kallikrein,* and are subsequently rapidly degraded into inactive fragments by various tissue kinases. Like histamine, bradykinin and kallidin are thought to be involved in the vascular responses associated with tissue injury and immune reactions. The kinins stimulate nocioceptive nerves and may thus be involved in the pain associated with tissue injury.

Transmural Pressure   In Chap. 7, we discussed the passive elastic mechanical properties of arteries and veins and how changes in transmural pressure affect their diameters. The effect of transmural pressure on arteriolar diameter is more complex because arterioles respond both passively *and actively* to changes in transmural pressure. For example, a sudden increase in the internal pressure within an arteriole produces (1) first an initial slight passive mechanical distention (slight because arterioles are relatively thick-walled and muscular), and (2) then an active constriction that, within seconds, may completely reverse the initial distention. A sudden decrease in transmural pressure elicits essentially the opposite response; i.e., an immediate passive decrease in diameter followed shortly by a decrease in active tone which returns the arteriolar diameter to near that which existed before the pressure change. The active phase of such behavior is referred to as a *myogenic response* because it seems to originate within the smooth muscle itself. The mechanism of the myogenic response is not known for certain, but stretch-sensitive ion channels on arteriolar vascular smooth muscle cells are likely candidates for involvement.

All arterioles have some normal distending pressure to which they probably are actively reacting. As we have previously alluded, the myogenic mechanism is therefore likely to be a fundamentally important factor in determining the basal tone of arterioles everywhere. Also, for obvious reasons and as will be soon discussed, the myogenic response is thought to be involved in the vascular reaction to any cardiovascular disturbance that involves a change in arteriolar transmural pressure.

Flow Responses Caused by Local Mechanisms   In organs with a highly variable metabolic rate, such as skeletal and cardiac muscle, the blood flow closely follows the tissue's metabolic rate. For example, skeletal muscle blood flow increases within seconds of the onset of muscle exercise and returns to control values shortly after exercise ceases. This phenomenon, which is illustrated in Fig. 8-3A, is known as *exercise* or *active hyperemia* (*hyperemia* means high flow). It should be clear how active hyperemia could result from the local metabolic vasodilator feedback on arteriolar smooth muscle.

   Reactive or postocclusion hyperemia is a higher than normal blood flow which occurs transiently after the removal of any restriction which has caused a

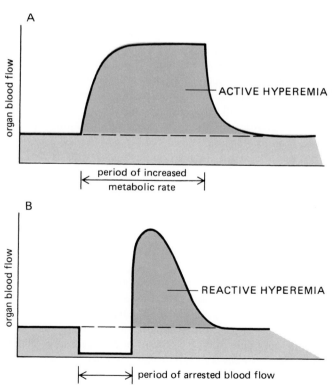

Figure 8-3   Organ blood flow responses caused by local mechanisms: active and reactive hyperemia.

period of lower than normal blood flow. The phenomenon is illustrated in Fig. 8-3*B*. For example, flow through an extremity is higher than normal for a period after a tourniquet is removed from the extremity. Both local metabolic and myogenic mechanisms may be involved in producing reactive hyperemia. The magnitude and duration of reactive hyperemia depend on the duration and severity of the occlusion as well as the metabolic rate of the tissue. These findings are best explained by an interstitial accumulation of metabolic vasodilator substances during the period of flow restriction. However, unexpectedly large flow increases can follow arterial occlusions lasting only 1 or 2 s. These may be explained best by a myogenic dilation response to the reduced intravascular pressure and decreased stretch of the arteriolar walls that exists during the period of occlusion.

Except when displaying active and reactive hyperemia, nearly all organs tend to keep their blood flow constant despite variations in arterial pressure— i.e., they *autoregulate* blood flow. As shown in Fig. 8-4*A*, an abrupt increase in arterial pressure is normally accompanied by an initial abrupt increase in organ blood flow which then gradually returns toward normal despite the sustained elevation in arterial pressure. The initial rise in flow with increased pressure is expected from the basic flow equation $(\dot{Q} = \Delta P/R)$. The subsequent return of flow toward the normal level is caused by a gradual increase in active arteriolar tone and resistance to blood flow. Ultimately a new steady state is reached with only slightly elevated blood flow because the increased driving pressure is counteracted by a higher than normal vascular resistance. As with the phenomenon of reactive hyperemia, blood flow autoregulation may be caused by both local metabolic feedback mechanisms and myogenic mechanisms. The arteriolar vasoconstriction responsible for the autoregulatory response shown in Fig. 8-4*A*, for example, may be partially due to (1) a "washout" of metabolic vasodilator factors from the interstitium by the excessive initial blood flow and (2) to a myogenic increase in arteriolar tone stimulated by the increase in stretching forces which the increase in pressure imposes on the vessel walls. There is also a *tissue pressure hypothesis* of blood flow autoregulation for which it is assumed that an abrupt increase in arterial pressure causes transcapillary fluid filtration and thus leads to a gradual increase in interstitial fluid volume and pressure. Presumably the increase in extravascular pressure would cause a decrease in vessel diameter by simple compression. This mechanism might be especially important in organs such as the kidney and brain whose volumes are constrained by external structures.

Although not illustrated in Fig. 8-4*A*, autoregulatory mechanisms operate in the opposite direction in response to a decrease in arterial pressure below the normal value. One important general consequence of local autoregulatory mechanisms is that the steady state blood flow in many organs tends to remain near the normal value over quite a wide range of arterial pressure. This is illustrated in the graph of Fig. 8-4*B*. As we shall discuss later, the inherent ability of certain organs to maintain adequate blood flow despite lower than normal arterial pressure is of considerable importance in situations such as shock from blood loss.

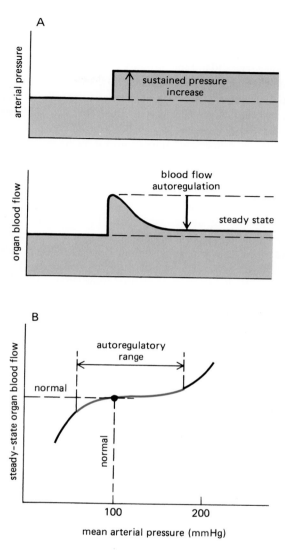

Figure 8-4 Autoregulation of organ blood flow.

Neural Influences on Arterioles

Sympathetic Vasoconstrictor Fibers   These neural fibers innervate arterioles in all systemic organs and provide by far the most important means of *reflex* control of the vasculature. These nerves release norepinephrine from their terminal structures in amounts generally proportional to their electrical activity.[2,3] Norepinephrine causes an increase in the tone of arterioles after combining with an *α-adrenergic receptor* on smooth muscle cells. Norepinephrine appears to increase vascular tone primarily by pharmacomechanical means. The mechanism involves G protein linkage of $α$-adrenergic receptors to phospholipase C and subsequent Ca^{2+} release from intracellular stores by the action of the second messenger IP_3, as was illustrated in the pharmacomechanical section of Fig. 8-1.

Sympathetic vasoconstrictor nerves normally have a continual or *tonic firing activity.* This tonic activity of sympathetic vasoconstrictor nerves makes the normal contractile tone of arterioles considerably greater than their basal tone. The additional component of vascular tone is called *neurogenic tone.* When the firing rate of sympathetic vasoconstrictor nerves is increased above normal, arterioles constrict and cause organ blood flow to fall below normal. Conversely, vasodilation and increased organ blood flow can be caused by sympathetic vasoconstrictor nerves if their normal tonic activity level is reduced. Thus an organ's blood flow can either be reduced below normal or be increased above normal by changes in the sympathetic vasoconstrictor fiber firing rate.

Other Neural Influences   Blood vessels, as a general rule, do not receive innervation from the parasympathetic division of the autonomic nervous system. However, *parasympathetic vasodilator nerves,* which release *acetylcholine,* are present in the vessels of the brain and the heart but their influence on arteriolar tone in these organs appears to be inconsequential. Parasympathetic vasodilator nerves are also present in the vessels of the salivary glands, pancreas, gastric mucosa, and external genitalia. In the latter, they are responsible for the vasodilation of inflow vessels responsible for erection.

Hormonal Influences on Arterioles

Under normal circumstances hormonal influences on blood vessels are generally thought to be of minor consequence in comparison to the local metabolic and neural influences. However, it should be emphasized that our understanding of how the cardiovascular system operates in many situations is incomplete. Thus, the hormones discussed below may play more important roles in cardiovascular regulation than we now appreciate.

[2]   Pharmacological studies indicate that the amount of norepinephrine released from sympathetic nerves at a given level of electrical activity can be modulated by presynaptic influences from a variety of agents. Norepinephrine release from sympathetic nerves is inhibited by high extracellular K^+, adenosine, certain prostaglandins, acetylcholine, and by norepinephrine itself. Angiotensin can enhance norepinephrine release from sympathetic nerves. Whether such effects are important in physiological situations is unclear at present.

[3]   In addition to norepinephrine, sympathetic vasoconstrictor nerves to some tissues are now thought to also release some ATP and neuropeptide Y as "co-transmitters." Like norepinephrine, these agents promote vessel constriction.

Circulating Catecholamines During activation of the sympathetic nervous system, the adrenal glands release the catecholamines *epinephrine* and *norepinephrine* into the bloodstream. Under normal circumstances, the blood levels of these agents are probably not high enough to cause significant cardiovascular effects. However, circulating catecholamines may have cardiovascular effects in situations (such as vigorous exercise or hemorrhagic shock) that involve high activity of the sympathetic nervous system. In general, the cardiovascular effects of high levels of circulating catecholamines parallel the direct effects of sympathetic activation which we have already discussed; both epinephrine and norepinephrine can activate cardiac β-adrenergic receptors to increase heart rate and myocardial contractility and can activate vascular α receptors to cause vasoconstriction. In addition to the α receptors that mediate vasoconstriction, arterioles in many organs also possess β-adrenergic receptors which mediate vasodilation.[4] Vascular β receptors are more sensitive to epinephrine than are vascular α receptors, so low levels of circulating epinephrine can cause vasodilation whereas higher levels cause α receptor-mediated vasoconstriction. Vascular β receptors are not innervated and therefore *not* activated by norepinephrine released from sympathetic vasoconstrictor nerves. The functional importance of these vascular β receptors is unclear since adrenal epinephrine release occurs during periods of increased sympathetic activity when arterioles would simultaneously be undergoing direct neurogenic vasoconstriction.

Vasopressin This polypeptide hormone, also known as antidiuretic hormone (ADH), plays an important role in extracellular fluid homeostasis and is released into the bloodstream from the posterior pituitary gland in response to low extracellular volume and/or high extracellular fluid osmolarity. Vasopressin acts on collecting ducts in the kidneys to decrease renal excretion of water. Its role in body fluid balance has some very important indirect influences on cardiovascular function which will be discussed in more detail in Chap. 10. Vasopressin, however, is also a potent arteriolar vasoconstrictor. While it is not thought to be significantly involved in normal vascular control, direct vascular constriction from abnormally high levels of vasopressin may be important in the response to certain disturbances such as severe blood loss through hemorrhage.

Angiotensin II Angiotensin II is a circulating polypeptide that regulates aldosterone release from the adrenal cortex as part of the system for controlling body sodium balance. This system, to be discussed in greater detail in Chap. 10, is very important in blood volume regulation. Angiotensin II is also a very potent vasoconstrictor agent. Although it should not be viewed as a normal regulator of arteriolar tone, direct vasoconstriction from angiotensin II seems to be an important component of the general cardiovascular response to severe blood loss. There is also strong evidence suggesting that direct vascular actions of angiotensin II may be involved in

---

[4] Vascular β receptors are labeled β_2 receptors and they can be distinguished pharmacologically from cardiac β receptors which are known as β_1 receptors.

intrarenal mechanisms for controlling kidney function. In addition, angiotensin II may be partially responsible for the abnormal vasoconstriction that accompanies many forms of hypertension. Again it should be emphasized that our knowledge of many pathological situations—including hypertension—is incomplete. These situations may well involve vascular influences which are not yet recognized.

CONTROL OF VENOUS TONE

Before considering the details of the control of venous tone, recall that venules and veins play a much different role in the cardiovascular system than do arterioles. Arterioles are the inflow valves that control the rate of nutritive blood flow through organs and individual regions within them. Appropriately, arterioles are usually strongly influenced by the current local metabolic needs of the region in which they reside, whereas veins are not. Veins do, however, collectively regulate the distribution of available blood volume between the peripheral and central venous pools. Recall that central blood volume (and therefore pressure) has a marked influence on stroke volume and cardiac output. Consequently, when one considers what *peripheral* veins are doing, one should be thinking primarily about what the effects will be on *central* venous pressure and cardiac output.

Veins contain vascular smooth muscle that is influenced by many of the things that influence vascular smooth muscle of arterioles. Constriction of the veins (venoconstriction) is largely mediated through activity of the sympathetic nerves that innervate them. As in arterioles, these sympathetic nerves release norepinephrine, which interacts with α receptors and produces an increase in venous tone and a decrease in vessel diameter. There are, however, several functionally important differences between veins and arterioles. Compared to arterioles, veins normally have little basal tone. Thus veins are normally in a vasodilated state. One important consequence of the lack of basal venous tone is that vasodilator metabolites that may accumulate in the tissue have little effect on veins.

Because of their thin walls, veins are much more susceptible to physical influences than are arterioles. The large effect of internal venous pressure on venous diameter was discussed in Chap. 7 and is evident in the pooling of blood in the veins of the lower extremities that occurs during prolonged standing (as will be discussed further in Chap. 11). Recall that changes in arteriolar resistance cause pressure changes in the vessels downstream of arterioles (Fig. 7-6) and, because of this, arteriolar tone can have an indirect effect on venous diameter. Arteriolar constriction tends to reduce venous pressure and thus decrease venous diameter. Arteriolar dilation has the opposite influence on venous diameter.

Often external compressional forces are an important determinant of venous volume. This is especially true of veins in skeletal muscle. Very high pressures are developed inside skeletal muscle tissue during contraction and cause venous vessels to collapse. Because veins and venules have one-way valves, the blood displaced from veins during skeletal muscle contraction is forced in the forward direction toward the right heart. In fact, rhythmic skeletal muscle contractions can produce a considerable pumping action, often called the *skeletal muscle pump,* which helps return blood to the heart during exercise.

SUMMARY OF PRIMARY VASCULAR CONTROL MECHANISMS

Vessels are subject to a wide variety of influences and special influences often apply to particular organs. Certain general factors, however, dominate the control of the peripheral vasculature when it is viewed from the standpoint of overall cardiovascular system function; these influences are summarized in Fig. 8-5. Basal tone, local metabolic vasodilator factors, and sympathetic vasoconstrictor nerves acting through α receptors are the major factors controlling arteriolar tone and therefore the blood flow rate through peripheral organs. Sympathetic vasoconstrictor nerves, internal pressure, and external compressional forces are

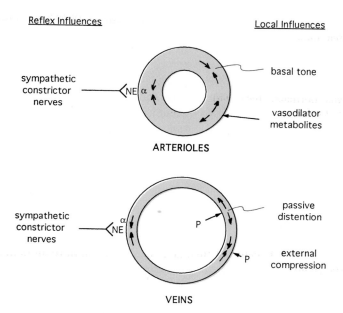

Figure 8-5 Primary influences on arterioles and veins. NE, norepinephrine; α, alpha-adrenergic receptor; P, pressure.

the most important influences on venous diameter and therefore peripheral organ blood volume.

VASCULAR CONTROL IN SPECIFIC ORGANS

As will become evident in the remaining sections of this chapter, the details of vascular control vary from organ to organ. However, with regard to flow control, most organs can be placed somewhere in a spectrum that ranges from almost total dominance by local metabolic mechanisms to almost total dominance by sympathetic nerves. The important general functional differences in methods of flow control between organs at the extremes of this spectrum are illustrated in Fig. 8-6.

In organs such as the brain, heart muscle, and skeletal muscle the normal organ blood flow is well below the maximum possible flow because the organs' normal resting arteriolar tone is high, as illustrated in Fig. 8-6A. Usually the normal blood flow is not greatly in excess of that required to meet the normal metabolic demands of the tissue. As shown in Fig. 8-6A, changes in the activity of sympathetic vasoconstrictor fibers have much less effect on blood flow to these organs than do changes in their metabolic rate. Increasing sympathetic vasoconstrictor fiber activity does tend to reduce flow by causing vasoconstriction, but this also causes a build-up of tissue metabolic vasodilators, which counteract the vasoconstriction and limit the extent of the flow reduction. Decreasing sympathetic vasoconstrictor fiber activity, in contrast, can cause only a modest increase in flow in these organs since their basal arteriolar tone is high. Increasing the tissue's metabolic rate and production of metabolically related vasodilator substances, however, can cause a large increase in flow by removing the normally high arteriolar tone.

A much different situation exists in the kidney, skin, and the splanchnic organs, as illustrated in Fig. 8-6B. The normal flow in these organs is relatively high and usually well in excess of the minimum required for tissue metabolism, and consequently the tissue concentrations of metabolically related vasodilator substances are very low. As indicated in Fig. 8-6B, increases in sympathetic vasoconstrictor fiber activity cause large reductions in flow to these organs. In part, this is because the normal arteriolar tone is substantially less than the maximum possible arteriolar tone and because sympathetic vasoconstriction is not strongly counteracted by local metabolic vasodilation in these organs. Usually even the reduced blood flow accompanying sympathetic vasoconstriction is sufficient to supply the tissue's basic metabolic needs. However, such reductions in blood flow may well curtail whatever blood-reconditioning function the organ in question performs and, while tolerated temporarily, cannot last indefinitely. As shown in Fig. 8-6B, blood flow in these organs increases to near its maximum possible value in the absence of sympathetic nerve activity. This indicates that arterioles in these organs have little basal tone. However, increasing metabolic rate in these organs has very little effect on blood flow since the normally high blood flow rate prevents metabolic vasodilator substances from accumulating to

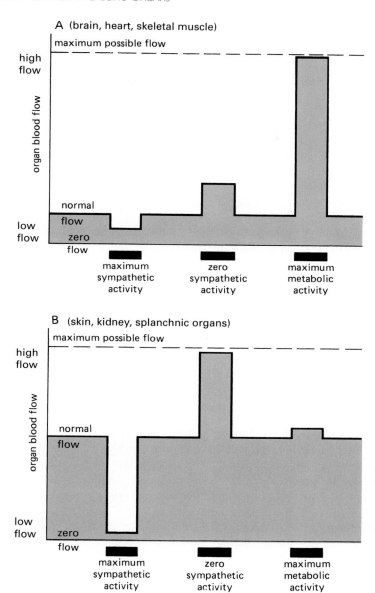

Figure 8-6 Blood flow responses in an organ with strong local metabolic control of arteriolar tone (A) and in an organ with strong neurogenic control of arteriolar tone (B).

the tissue concentrations required to affect arteriolar tone. Organs in which blood flow is regulated predominantly by sympathetic nerves participate to a great extent in the cardiovascular reflex responses that will be discussed in Chaps. 10 and 11.

Coronary Blood Flow

The major right and left coronary arteries that serve the heart tissue are the first vessels to branch off the aorta. Thus the driving force for myocardial blood flow is the systemic arterial pressure, just as it is for other systemic organs. Most of the blood that flows through the myocardial tissue returns to the right atrium by way of a large cardiac vein called the coronary sinus.

Local Metabolic Control As emphasized before, coronary blood flow is controlled primarily by local metabolic mechanisms and thus it responds rapidly and accurately to changes in myocardial oxygen consumption. In a resting individual, the myocardium extracts 70 to 75 percent of the oxygen in the blood that passes through it. Coronary sinus blood normally has a lower oxygen content than blood at any other place in the cardiovascular system. Myocardial oxygen extraction cannot increase significantly from its resting value. Consequently, increases in myocardial oxygen consumption must be accompanied by appropriate increases in coronary blood flow. In fact, coronary blood flow normally follows myocardial oxygen consumption so closely that the oxygen levels in coronary sinus blood are essentially constant regardless of the rate of myocardial oxygen consumption.

The issue of which metabolic vasodilator factors play the dominant role in modulating the tone of coronary arterioles is unresolved at present. Many believe that adenosine, released from myocardial muscle cells in response to insufficient supplies of oxygen, may be an important local coronary metabolic vasodilator influence. Regardless of the specific details, myocardial oxygen consumption is the most important influence on coronary blood flow.

Systolic Compression Large forces and/or pressures are generated *within* the myocardial tissue during cardiac muscle contraction. Such intramyocardial forces press on the outside of coronary vessels and cause them to collapse during systole. Because of this *systolic compression* and the associated collapse of coronary vessels, coronary vascular resistance is greatly increased during systole. The result, at least for much of the left ventricular myocardium, is that coronary flow is lower during systole than during diastole, even though systemic arterial pressure (i.e., coronary perfusion pressure) is highest during systole. This is illustrated in the left coronary artery flow trace shown in Fig. 8-7. Systolic compression has much less effect on flow through the right ventricular myocardium, as is evident from the right coronary artery flow trace in Fig. 8-7. This is because the peak systolic intraventricular pressure is much lower for the right heart than

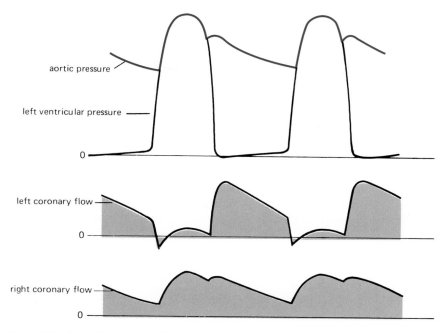

Figure 8-7 Phasic flows in the left and right coronary arteries in relation to aortic and left ventricular pressures.

for the left, and the systolic compressional forces in the right ventricular wall are correspondingly less than those in the left ventricular wall.

Systolic compressional forces on coronary vessels are greater in the endocardial (inside) layers of the left ventricular wall than in the epicardial layers.[5] Thus the flow to the endocardial layers of the left ventricle is impeded more than the flow to epicardial layers by systolic compression. Normally the endocardial region of the myocardium can make up for the lack of flow during systole by a high flow in the diastolic interval. However, when coronary blood flow is limited — for example, by coronary disease and stenosis — the endocardial layers of the left ventricle are often the first regions of the heart to have difficulty maintaining a flow sufficient for their metabolic needs. *Myocardial infarcts* (areas of tissue killed by lack of blood flow) occur most frequently in the endocardial layers of the left ventricle.

---

[5] Consider that the endocardial surface of the left ventricle is exposed to intraventricular pressure (≈ 120 mmHg during systole), while the epicardial surface is exposed only to intrathoracic pressure (≈ 0 mm Hg).

Neural Influences on Coronary Flow   Coronary arterioles are densely innervated with sympathetic vasoconstrictor fibers, yet when the activity of the sympathetic nervous system increases, the coronary arterioles normally vasodilate
rather than vasoconstrict. This is because an increase in sympathetic tone increases myocardial oxygen consumption by increasing heart rate and contractility. The increased local metabolic vasodilator influence apparently outweighs
the concurrent vasoconstrictor influence due to an increase in the activity of
sympathetic vasoconstrictor fibers that terminate on coronary arterioles. It has
been experimentally demonstrated that a given increase in cardiac sympathetic
nerve activity causes a greater increase in coronary blood flow after the direct
vasoconstrictor influence of sympathetic nerves on coronary vessels has been
eliminated with α-receptor blocking agents. However, sympathetic vasoconstrictor nerves do not appear to influence coronary flow enough to affect the mechanical performance of normal hearts. Whether these coronary vasoconstrictor fibers
might be functionally important in certain pathological situations is an open
question.

As mentioned previously, coronary arterioles also receive parasympathetic
vasodilator fiber innervation. However, their role in the normal control of coronary blood flow appears to be inconsequential.

Skeletal Muscle Blood Flow

Collectively, the skeletal muscles constitute 40 to 45 percent of body weight—
more than any other single body organ. Even at rest, about 15 percent of the cardiac output goes to skeletal muscle, and during strenuous exercise skeletal muscle may receive up to 70 percent of the cardiac output. Thus skeletal muscle
blood flow is an important factor in overall cardiovascular hemodynamics.

Because of the high level of intrinsic tone of the resistance vessels in resting skeletal muscles, the blood flow per gram of tissue is quite low when compared to that of other organs such as the kidneys. However, resting skeletal muscle blood flow is still substantially above that required to sustain its metabolic
needs. Resting skeletal muscles normally extract only 25 to 30 percent of the
oxygen delivered to them in arterial blood. Changes in the activity of sympathetic vasoconstrictor fibers do alter resting muscle blood flow. For example,
maximum sympathetic discharge rates can decrease blood flow in a resting muscle to less than one-fourth its normal value, and conversely, if all neurogenic
tone is removed, resting skeletal muscle blood flow may double. This is a modest increase in flow compared to the 20-fold increase in flow that can occur in an
exercising skeletal muscle. Nonetheless, because of the large mass of tissue involved, changes in the vascular resistance of resting skeletal muscle brought
about by changes in sympathetic activity are very important in the overall reflex
regulation of arterial pressure.

A particularly important characteristic of skeletal muscle is its very wide
range of metabolic rates. During heavy exercise the oxygen consumption rate of
and oxygen extraction by skeletal muscle tissue can reach the high values typical

of the myocardium. In most respects, the factors that control blood flow to exercising muscle are similar to those that control coronary blood flow. Local metabolic control of arteriolar tone is very strong in exercising skeletal muscle, and muscle oxygen consumption is the most important determinant of blood flow in exercising skeletal muscle.

As will be discussed in Chap. 11, the cardiovascular response to muscle exercise involves a general increase in sympathetic activity. A given increase in sympathetic nerve activity causes a much smaller relative (percentage) decrease in the blood flow to exercising muscle than to resting muscle. Thus, it is believed that exercise somehow inhibits the influence of sympathetic nerves on arteriolar tone in skeletal muscle. In part, this is explained by the presence of strong local metabolic vasodilator influences on arterioles in exercising muscle. Also, local increases in H^+, K^+, osmolarity, and adenosine may depress norepinephrine release from sympathetic nerve terminals during exercise. The fact remains, however, that the general increase in sympathetic activity that normally occurs with physical exertion does restrain, to some extent, the degree of local metabolic vasodilation that occurs in the active muscles. This does not appear to adversely affect muscle performance during submaximal efforts, but maximum muscle blood flow, oxygen consumption rate, and performance are reduced by sympathetic activation.

As in the heart, muscle contraction produces large compressional forces within the tissue, which can collapse vessels and impede blood flow. Strong, sustained (tetanic) skeletal muscle contractions may actually stop muscle blood flow. About 10 percent of the total blood volume is normally contained within the veins of skeletal muscle, and during rhythmic exercise the "skeletal muscle pump" is very effective in displacing blood from skeletal muscle veins. Blood displaced from skeletal muscle into the central venous pool is an important factor in the hemodynamics of strenuous whole body exercise.

The veins in skeletal muscle are rather sparsely innervated with sympathetic vasoconstrictor fibers, and the rather small volume of blood that can be mobilized from skeletal muscle by sympathetic nerve activation is probably not of much significance to total body hemodynamics. This is in sharp contrast to the large displacement of blood from exercising muscle by the muscle pump mechanism.

Cerebral Blood Flow

Adequate cerebral blood flow is of paramount importance for survival because unconsciousness occurs very rapidly after an interruption in flow. One rule of overall cardiovascular system function is that, in *all* situations, measures are taken that are appropriate to preserve adequate blood flow to the brain.

The brain as a whole has a nearly constant rate of metabolism that, on a per gram basis, is nearly as high as that of myocardial tissue. Cerebral blood flow appears to be regulated almost entirely by local mechanisms. Flow through the cerebrum is autoregulated very strongly and is little affected by changes in arterial pressure unless if falls below about 60 mmHg. When arterial pressure decreases below 60 mmHg, brain blood flow decreases proportionately. It is presently unresolved whether metabolic mechanisms or myogenic mechanisms or both are involved in the phenomenon of cerebral autoregulation.

Presumably because the overall average metabolic rate of brain tissue shows little variation, total brain blood flow is remarkably constant over nearly all situations. The cerebral activity in discrete locations within the brain, however, changes from situation to situation. As a result, blood flow to discrete regions is not constant but closely follows the local neuronal activity. The mechanisms responsible for this strong local control of cerebral blood flow are as yet undefined, but H^+, K^+, O_2, and adenosine seem most likely to be involved.

Cerebral blood flow does increase whenever the partial pressure of carbon dioxide (P_{CO_2}) is raised above normal in the arterial blood. Conversely, cerebral blood flow decreases whenever arterial blood P_{CO_2} falls below normal. It appears that cerebral arterioles respond not to changes in P_{CO_2} but to changes in the extracellular H^+ concentration (i.e., pH) caused by changes in P_{CO_2}. Cerebral arterioles also vasodilate whenever the partial pressure of oxygen (P_{O_2}) in arterial blood falls significantly below normal values. Higher than normal arterial blood P_{O_2}, such as that caused by oxygen inhalation, produces only a slight decrease in cerebral blood flow.

Although cerebral vessels receive both sympathetic vasoconstrictor and parasympathetic vasodilator fiber innervation, cerebral blood flow is influenced very little by changes in the activity of either under normal circumstances. Sympathetic vasoconstrictor responses do, however, seem important in protecting cerebral vessels from excessive passive distention following large, abrupt increases in arterial pressure.

Brain capillaries are unique in that they are considerably less porous than those in other organs, and they greatly restrict the transcapillary movement of polar particles. The diffusional restriction and other specific metabolic mechanisms associated with the endothelial cells of brain capillaries constitute what is known as the *blood-brain barrier*.[6] Because of the blood-brain barrier, the extracellular space of the brain represents a special fluid compartment in which the chemical composition is regulated separately from that in the plasma and general body extracellular fluid compartment. The extracellular compartment of the brain encompasses both interstitial fluid and *cerebrospinal fluid* (CSF) which surrounds the brain and spinal cord and fills the brain ventricles. The CSF is formed from plasma by selective secretion (not simple filtration) by specialized tissues, the *choroid plexes*, located within the ventricles. These processes regulate the chemical composition of the CSF. The interstitial fluid of the brain takes on the chemical composition of CSF through free diffusional exchange.

The blood-brain barrier serves to protect the cerebral cells from ionic disturbances in the plasma. Also, by exclusion and/or endothelial cell metabolism,

---

[6] Brain capillaries have a special carrier system for glucose and present no barrier to O_2 and CO_2 diffusion. Thus, the blood-brain barrier does not restrict nutrient supply to the brain tissue.

it prevents circulating hormones (and many drugs) from influencing the parenchymal cells of the brain and the vascular smooth muscle cells in brain vessels.

Splanchnic Blood Flow

A number of abdominal organs, including the gastrointestinal tract, spleen, pancreas, and liver, are collectively supplied with what is called the *splanchnic blood flow*. Splanchnic blood flow is supplied to these abdominal organs through many arteries, but it all ultimately passes through the liver and returns to the inferior vena cava through the hepatic veins.

The organs of the splanchnic region receive about 25 percent of the resting cardiac output and moreover contain more than 20 percent of the circulating blood volume. Thus adjustments in either the blood flow or the blood volume of this region have extremely important effects on the cardiovascular system.

There is a great diversity of function among individual organs and even regions within organs in the splanchnic region. Blood flow is required to support secretory and absorptive processes as well as muscular contractions of the gastrointestinal tract. The mechanisms of vascular control in specific areas of the splanchnic region are not well understood but are likely to be quite varied. Nonetheless, since most of the splanchnic organs are involved in the digestion and absorption of food from the gastrointestinal tract, splanchnic blood flow increases after food ingestion. A large meal can elicit a 30 to 100 percent increase in splanchnic flow, but individual organs in the splanchnic region probably have higher percentage increases in flow at certain times because they are involved sequentially in the digestion-absorption process.

Collectively, the splanchnic organs have a relatively high blood flow and extract only 15 to 20 percent of the oxygen delivered to them in the arterial blood. In general, the situation of Fig. 8-6B applies to the splanchnic bed and the sympathetic nerves play a significant role in vascular control. The arteries and veins of all the organs involved in the splanchnic circulation are richly innervated with sympathetic vasoconstrictor nerves. Maximal activation of sympathetic vasoconstrictor nerves can produce an 80 percent reduction in flow to the splanchnic region and also cause a large shift of blood from the splanchnic organs to the central venous pool. In humans, a large fraction of the blood mobilized from the splanchnic circulation during periods of sympathetic activation comes from the constriction of veins in the liver. In many other species, the spleen acts as a major reservoir from which blood is mobilized by sympathetically mediated contraction of smooth muscle located in the outer capsule of the organ.

Renal Blood Flow

The kidneys normally receive approximately 20 percent of the cardiac output of a resting individual, and since this can be reduced to practically zero, the control of renal blood *flow* is important to overall cardiovascular control. However, because the kidneys are such small organs, changes in renal blood *volume* are inconsequential to overall cardiovascular hemodynamics.

Although the renal vascular bed is specialized in many ways that are important to renal function (e.g., two distinct capillary beds arranged in series), renal blood flow follows the patterns of adjustment shown in Fig. 8-6B well. Increases in sympathetic vasoconstrictor activity can markedly reduce total renal blood flow by increasing the neurogenic tone of renal resistance vessels. In fact, extreme situations involving intense and prolonged sympathetic vasoconstrictor activity can lead to renal failure.

The renal vascular resistance adjusts to keep renal blood flow nearly constant over a wide range of arterial pressures—i.e., the kidneys autoregulate strongly. The mechanism responsible for the autoregulation of renal blood flow has not been established. Myogenic, tissue pressure, and metabolic hypotheses have all been advanced. However, it is difficult to imagine how strong local metabolic feedback could exist in an organ with blood flow normally greatly in excess of the tissue's metabolic needs. The fact that the renal circulation shows little or no reactive hyperemia also argues against a significant influence of local vasodilator metabolites on renal arterioles.

The mechanisms responsible for the intrinsic regulation of renal blood flow and kidney function have not been established. While studies suggest that prostaglandins and some intrarenal renin-angiotensin system may be involved, the whole issue of local renal vascular control remains quite obscure. Renal function is itself of paramount importance to overall cardiovascular function, as will be described in Chap. 10.

Cutaneous Blood Flow

The metabolic activity of body cells produces heat, which must be lost in order for the body temperature to remain constant. The skin is the primary site of exchange of body heat with the external environment. Alterations in cutaneous blood flow in response to various metabolic states and environmental conditions provide the primary mechanism responsible for temperature homeostasis. (Other mechanisms such as shivering, sweating, and panting also participate in body temperature regulation under more extreme conditions.)

Cutaneous blood flow, which is about 6 percent of the resting cardiac output, can decrease to about one-twentieth of its normal value when heat is to be retained (e.g., in a cold environment, during the development stages of a fever). In contrast, cutaneous blood flow can increase up to seven times its normal value when heat is to be lost (e.g., in a hot environment, accompanying a high metabolic rate, after a fever breaks).

The anatomic interconnections between microvessels in the skin are highly specialized and extremely complex. An extensive system of interconnected veins called the *venous plexus* normally contains the largest fraction of cutaneous blood volume, which, in individuals with lightly pigmented skin, gives the skin a reddish hue. To a large extent, heat transfer from the blood takes place across the large surface area of the venous plexus. The venous plexus is richly innervated with sympathetic vasoconstrictor nerves. When these fibers are activated, blood is displaced from the venous plexus, and this helps reduce heat loss and also lightens the skin color. Since the skin is one of the largest body organs, venous constriction can shift a considerable amount of blood into the central venous pool.

Cutaneous resistance vessels are also richly innervated with sympathetic vasoconstrictor nerves, and since these fibers have a normal tonic activity, cutaneous resistance vessels normally have a high degree of neurogenic tone. In general, cutaneous blood flow follows the response patterns shown in Fig. 8-6B. When body temperature rises above normal, skin blood flow is increased by reflex mechanisms. In certain areas (such as the hands, ears, and nose) vasodilation appears to result entirely from the withdrawal of sympathetic vasoconstrictor tone. In other areas (such as the forearm, forehead, chin, neck, and chest) the cutaneous vasodilation that occurs with body heating greatly exceeds that which occurs with just the removal of sympathetic vasoconstrictor tone. This "active" vasodilation is closely linked to the onset of sweating in these areas. The sweat glands in human cutaneous tissue are innervated by *cholinergic sympathetic fibers* that release acetylcholine. Activation of these nerves elicit sweating *and* an associated marked cutaneous vasodilation. The exact mechanism for this sweating-related cutaneous vasodilation remains unclear because it is not abolished by agents which block acetylcholine's vascular effects. It has long been thought that it was caused by local bradykinin formation secondary to the process of sweat gland activation. Evidence suggests that instead the cholinergic sympathetic nerves to sweat glands may release not only acetylcholine but also a nonadrenergic, noncholinergic (NANC) vasodilator cotransmitter that has yet to be identified. While these special sympathetic nerves are very important to temperature regulation, they do not participate in the normal, moment-to-moment, regulation of the cardiovascular system.

In addition to responding reflexly to changes in body temperature, cutaneous vessels also respond to local skin temperature. In general, local cooling leads to local vasoconstriction and local heating causes local vasodilation. The mechanisms for this are unknown. If the hand is placed in ice water, there is initially a nearly complete cessation of hand blood flow accompanied by intense pain. After some minutes, hand blood flow begins to rise to reach values greatly in excess of the normal value, hand temperature increases, and the pain disappears. This phenomenon is referred to as *cold-induced vasodilation*. With continued immersion, hand blood flow cycles every few minutes between periods of essentially no flow and periods of vasodilation. The mechanism responsible for cold vasodilation is unknown, but it has been suggested that norepinephrine may lose its ability to constrict vessels when their temperature approaches 0°C. Whatever the mechanism, cold-induced vasodilation apparently serves to protect exposed tissues from cold damage.

Tissue damage from burns, ultraviolet radiation, cold injury, caustic chemicals, and mechanical trauma produce reactions in skin blood flow. A classical reaction called the *triple response* is evoked after vigorously stroking the skin with a blunt point. The first component of the triple response is a *red line* that develops along the direct path of the abrasion in about 15 s. Shortly thereafter, an irregular *red flare* appears that extends about 2 cm on either side of the red line. Finally, after a minute or two, a *wheal* appears along the line of the injury. The mechanisms involved in the triple response are unknown, but it seems likely that histamine release from damaged cells is at least partially responsible for the dilation evidenced by the red line and the subsequent edema formation of the wheal. The red flare seems to involve nerves in some sort of a local *axon reflex* because it can be evoked immediately after cutaneous nerves are sectioned but not after the peripheral portions of the sectioned nerves degenerate.

Pulmonary Blood Flow

The rate of blood flow through the lungs is necessarily equal to cardiac output in all circumstances. When cardiac output increases threefold during exercise, for example, pulmonary blood flow must also increase threefold. Whereas the flow through a systemic organ is determined by its vascular resistance $(\dot{Q} = \Delta P/R)$, the blood flow rate through the lungs is determined simply by the cardiac output $(\dot{Q} = CO)$. Pulmonary vessels do, however, offer some vascular resistance. Although the level of pulmonary vascular resistance does not usually influence the pulmonary flow rate, it is important because it is one of the determinants of pulmonary arterial pressure $(\Delta P = \dot{Q} \cdot R)$. Recall that mean *pulmonary* arterial pressure is about 13 mmHg, whereas mean *systemic* arterial pressure is about 100 mmHg. The reason for the difference in pulmonary and systemic arterial pressures is not that the right heart is weaker than the left heart but rather that pulmonary vascular resistance is inherently much lower than systemic total peripheral resistance. The pulmonary bed has a low resistance because it has relatively large vessels throughout.

A very important distinction between the systemic and pulmonary arteries and arterioles is that the pulmonary vessels are less muscular and more compliant. When pulmonary arterial pressure increases, the pulmonary arteries and arterioles become larger in diameter. Thus an increase in pulmonary arterial pressure *decreases* pulmonary vascular resistance. This phenomenon is important because it tends to limit the increase in pulmonary arterial pressure which occurs with increases in cardiac output.

The most important active response in the pulmonary vasculature is the *hypoxic vasoconstriction* of pulmonary arterioles. Recall that systemic arterioles dilate in response to low P_{O_2}. The mechanisms that cause the opposite response in pulmonary vessels are unclear. Current evidence suggests that local prostaglandin synthesis may be involved in pulmonary hypoxic vasoconstriction. Whatever the mechanism, hypoxic vasoconstriction is essential to efficient lung gas exchange because it diverts blood flow away from areas of the lung which are underventilated. Consequently, the best-ventilated areas of the lung also receive the most blood flow. Presumably as a consequence of hypoxic arteriolar vasoconstriction, general hypoxia (such as that encountered at high altitude) causes an increase in pulmonary vascular resistance and pulmonary arterial hypertension.

Both pulmonary arteries and veins receive sympathetic vasoconstrictor fiber innervation, but reflex influences on pulmonary vessels appear to be much less important than the physical and local hypoxic influences. Pulmonary veins serve a blood reservoir function for the cardiovascular system, and sympathetic vasoconstriction of pulmonary veins may be important in mobilizing this blood during periods of general cardiovascular stress.

A consequence of the low mean pulmonary arterial pressure is the low pulmonary capillary hydrostatic pressure of about 8 mmHg (compared with 25 mmHg in systemic capillaries). Because the plasma oncotic pressure in lung capillaries is near 25 mmHg, as it is in all capillaries, it is tempting to conclude that the transcapillary forces in the lungs would strongly favor continual fluid reabsorption. This cannot be the case, however, since the lungs, like other tissues, continually produce some lymph; net capillary filtration is required to produce lymphatic fluid. This is possible despite the unusually low pulmonary capillary hydrostatic pressure because pulmonary interstitial fluid has an unusually high protein concentration and thus oncotic pressure.

Initiation of Pulmonary Circulation at Birth Fetal gas exchange occurs entirely in the placenta, and the fetal circulation completely bypasses the lungs. No blood flows into the pulmonary artery because the vascular resistance in the collapsed fetal lungs is essentially infinite. By the special arrangements shown in Fig. 8-8, the fetal right and left hearts actually operate in parallel to pump blood

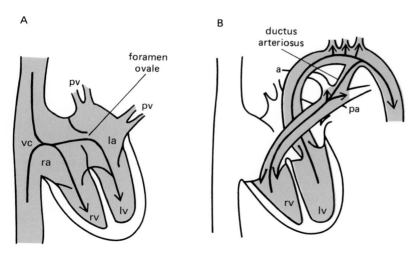

Figure 8-8 Fetal circulation during cardiac filling (A) and cardiac ejection (B); ra, right atrium; la, left atrium; rv, right ventricle; lv, left ventricle; vc, venae cavae; pv, pulmonary veins; a, aorta; pa, pulmonary artery.

through the systemic organs and the placenta. As shown in Fig. 8-8A, fetal blood returning from the systemic organs and placenta fills both the left and right hearts together because of an opening in the intraatrial septum called the *foramen ovale.* As indicated in Fig. 8-8B, blood that is pumped by the fetal right heart does not enter the occluded pulmonary circulation but rather is diverted into the aorta through a vascular connection between the pulmonary artery and the aorta called the *ductus arteriosis.*

An abrupt decrease in pulmonary vascular resistance occurs at birth with the onset of lung ventilation. This permits blood to begin flowing into the lungs from the pulmonary artery and tends to lower pulmonary arterial pressure. Meanwhile, total systemic vascular resistance increases greatly because of the interruption of flow through the placenta. This causes a rise in aortic pressure, which retards or even reverses the flow through the ductus arteriosis. Through mechanisms that are incompletely understood but clearly linked to a rise in blood oxygen tension, the ductus arteriosis gradually constricts and completely closes over a period normally ranging from hours to a few days. The circulatory changes that occur at birth tend to simultaneously increase the pressure afterload on the left heart and decrease that on the right. This indirectly causes left atrial pressure to increase above that in the right atrium so that the pressure gradient for flow through the foramen ovale is reversed. Reverse flow through the foramen ovale is, however, prevented by a flaplike valve that covers the opening in the left atrium. Normally, the foramen ovale eventually is closed permanently by the growth of fibrous tissue.

Study Questions: 35 to 41.

9

CENTRAL VENOUS PRESSURE AS AN INDICATOR OF CIRCULATORY STATUS

OBJECTIVES

The student understands how central venous pressure can be used to assess circulatory states and how venous return, cardiac output, and central venous pressure are interrelated:

1. Defines venous return and explains how it is distinguished from cardiac output.
2. States the reason why cardiac output and venous return must be equal in the steady state.
3. Lists the factors that control venous return.
4. Describes the relationship between venous return and central venous pressure and draws the normal venous return curve.
5. Defines peripheral venous pressure.
6. Lists the factors that determine peripheral venous pressure.
7. Predicts the shifts in the venous return curve that occur with altered blood volume and altered venous tone.
8. Describes how the output of the left heart pump is matched to that of the right heart pump.
9. Draws the normal venous return and cardiac output curves on a graph and describes the significance of the point of curve intersection.
10. Predicts how normal venous return, cardiac output, and central venous pressure will be altered with any given combination of changes in cardiac sympathetic tone, peripheral venous sympathetic tone, or circulating blood volume.
11. Identifies possible conditions that result in abnormally high or low central venous pressure.

Any adjustment made by a single component in the cardiovascular system produces hemodynamic alterations throughout the system. For example, an increase in peripheral venous tone usually results in increased cardiac output. In this chapter we will describe the interactions that occur between the heart and the peripheral vasculature at the connection between them on the venous side and how measures of central venous pressure can provide information about the circulatory system.

Recall that we have described a space, called the *central venous pool,* that corresponds roughly to the volume enclosed by the right atrium and the great veins in the thorax. Blood *leaves* the central venous pool by entering the right ventricle at a rate that is equal to the cardiac output. *Venous return,* in contrast, is by definition the rate at which blood returns to the thorax from the peripheral vascular beds and thus is the rate at which blood *enters* the central venous pool. The important distinction between venous return *to* the central venous pool and cardiac output *from* the central venous pool is illustrated in Fig. 9-1.

In any stable situation, venous return must equal cardiac output or blood would gradually accumulate in either the central venous pool or the peripheral vasculature. However, there often are temporary differences between cardiac output and venous return. Whenever such differences exist, the volume of the central venous pool must be changing. Since the central venous pool is enclosed by elastic tissues, any change in central venous volume produces a corresponding change in central venous pressure.

We discussed in Chap. 4 how any change in central venous pressure changes cardiac output (the Frank-Starling law of the heart). In this chapter, we will show how alterations in central venous pressure also change venous return. Thus, whenever an influence acts on the heart to change cardiac output, a change in central venous pressure is automatically produced that causes an appropriate change in venous return. Conversely, whenever venous return is altered by a peripheral vascular influence, a change in central venous pressure is automatically produced which causes an appropriate adjustment in cardiac output. To appreciate these concepts more fully, we must first understand how central pressure influences venous return.

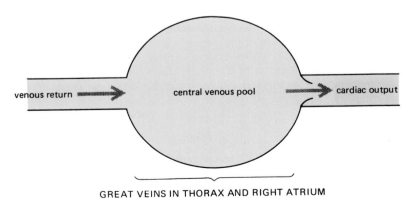

GREAT VEINS IN THORAX AND RIGHT ATRIUM

Figure 9-1   Distinction between cardiac output and venous return.

VENOUS RETURN CURVE

The important factors involved in the process of venous return can be summarized as shown in Fig. 9-2A. Basically, blood flows from the peripheral venous pool to the central venous pool through converging vessels. Anatomically the peripheral venous pool is scattered throughout the systemic organs, but functionally it can be viewed as a single vascular space that has a particular pressure (P_{PV}) at any instant of time. The blood flow rate between the peripheral venous pool and the central venous pool is governed by the basic flow equation ($\dot{Q} = \Delta P/R$), where ΔP is the pressure drop between the peripheral and central venous pools and R is the small resistance associated with the peripheral veins.

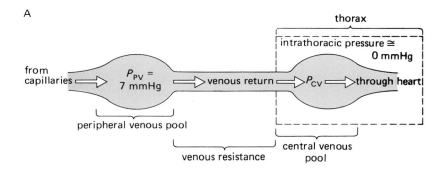

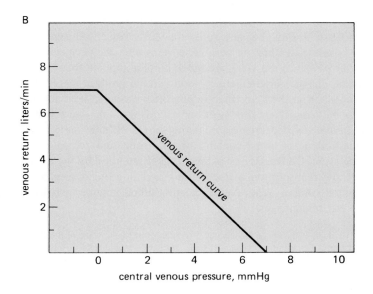

Figure 9-2   *A. Factors influencing venous return. B. The venous return curve.*

In the example of Fig. 9-2, peripheral venous pressure is assumed to be 7 mmHg. Thus there will be no venous return when the central venous pressure (P_{CV}) is also 7 mmHg. This situation is represented in the graph of Fig. 9-2*B* as the intersection of the venous return curve with the central venous pressure axis at 7 mmHg. If the peripheral venous pressure remains at 7 mmHg, then decreasing central venous pressure will increase the pressure drop across the venous resistance and consequently cause an increase in venous return. This relationship is summarized by the *venous return curve,* which shows how venous return increases as central venous pressure drops.[1] If central venous pressure reaches very low values and falls below the intrathoracic pressure, the veins in the thorax collapse and tend to limit venous return. In the example of Fig. 9-2, intrathoracic pressure is taken to be 0 mmHg and the flat portion of the venous return curve indicates that lowering central venous pressure below 0 mmHg produces no additional increase in venous return.

Just as a cardiac function curve shows how central venous pressure influences cardiac output, a venous return curve shows how central venous pressure influences venous return, if other factors remain constant.

INFLUENCE OF PERIPHERAL VENOUS PRESSURE ON VENOUS RETURN

As can be deduced from Fig. 9-2*A*, it is the pressure difference between the peripheral and central venous pools that determines venous return. Therefore, an increase in peripheral venous pressure can be just as effective in increasing venous return as a drop in central venous pressure.

The two ways in which peripheral venous pressure can change were discussed in Chap. 7. First, because veins are elastic vessels, changes in the *volume* of blood contained within the peripheral veins alter the peripheral venous pressure. Moreover, since the veins are much more compliant than any other vascular segment, changes in circulating blood volume produce larger changes in the volume of blood in the veins than in any other vascular segment. For example, blood loss by hemorrhage or loss of body fluids through severe sweating, vomiting, or diarrhea will decrease circulating blood volume and significantly decrease the volume of blood contained in the veins and decrease the peripheral venous pressure. Conversely, transfusion, fluid retention by the kidney, or transcapillary fluid reabsorption will increase circulating blood volume and increase venous blood volume. Whenever circulating blood volume increases, peripheral venous pressure increases.

---

[1]   The slope of the venous return curve is determined by the value of the venous vascular resistance. Lowering the venous vascular resistance would tend to raise the venous return curve and make it steeper because more venous return would result for a given difference between P_{PV} and P_{CV}. However, if P_{PV} is 7 mmHg, venous return will be zero when $P_{CV} = $ 7 mmHg at any level of venous vascular resistance ($\dot{Q} = \Delta P/R$). We have chosen to ignore the complicating issue of changes in venous vascular resistance because they do not affect the general conclusions to be drawn from the discussion of venous return curves.

Recall from Chap. 7 that the second way that peripheral venous pressure can be altered is through changes in venous tone produced by increasing or decreasing the activity of sympathetic vasoconstrictor nerves supplying the venous smooth muscle. Peripheral venous pressure increases whenever the activity of sympathetic vasoconstrictor fibers to veins increases. In addition, an increase in any force compressing veins from the outside has the same effect on the pressure inside veins as an increase in venous tone. Thus, such things as muscle exercise and wearing elastic stockings tend to increase peripheral venous pressure.

Whenever peripheral venous pressure is altered, the relationship between central venous pressure and venous return is also altered. For example, whenever peripheral venous pressure is increased by increases in blood volume or by sympathetic stimulation, the venous return curve shifts upward and to the right, as shown in Fig. 9-3. This relationship can be most easily understood by focusing first on the central venous pressure at which there will be no venous return. When peripheral venous pressure is 7 mmHg, venous return is zero when central venous pressure is 7 mmHg. When peripheral venous pressure is increased to 10 mmHg, considerable venous return occurs with a central venous pressure of 7 mmHg, and venous return stops only when central venous pressure is raised to 10 mmHg. Thus, increasing peripheral venous pressure shifts the whole venous return curve to the right. By similar logic, decreased peripheral venous pressure caused by blood loss or decreased sympathetic vasoconstriction of peripheral veins shifts the venous return curve to the left, as indicated in Fig. 9-3.

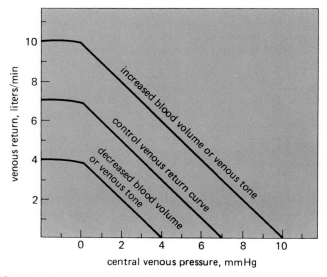

Figure 9-3   Effect of changes in blood volume and venous tone on venous return curves.

DETERMINATION OF CARDIAC OUTPUT AND VENOUS RETURN BY CENTRAL VENOUS PRESSURE

The significance of the fact that central venous pressure simultaneously affects both cardiac output and venous return can be best seen by plotting the cardiac output curve (the Frank-Starling curve) and the venous return curve on the same graph, as in Fig. 9-4.

Central venous pressure, as defined earlier, is the filling pressure of the right heart. Strictly speaking, this pressure directly affects only the stroke volume and output of the *right* heart pump. In most contexts, however, "cardiac output" implies the output of the *left* heart pump. How is it then, as has often been previously implied, that central venous pressure (the filling pressure of the right heart) profoundly affects cardiac output (the output of the left heart)? The short answer is that in the steady state, the right and left hearts have equal outputs. (Since the right and left hearts always beat with identical rates, this implies that their stroke volumes must be equal in the steady state.) The proper answer is that changes in central venous pressure automatically cause essentially parallel changes in the filling pressure of the left heart (i.e., in left atrial pressure). Consider, for example, the following sequence of consequences that a small stepwise increase in central venous pressure has on a heart that previously was in a steady state:

1 Increased central venous pressure.
2 Increased right ventricular stroke volume via Starling's law.

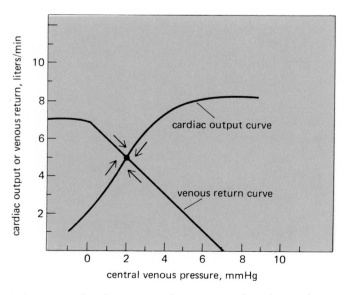

Figure 9-4   Interaction of cardiac output and venous return through central venous pressure.

3 Increased output of right heart.
4 Right heart output temporarily exceeds that of the left heart.
5 As long as this imbalance exists, blood accumulates in the pulmonary vasculature and raises pulmonary venous and left atrial pressure.
6 Increased left atrial pressure increases left ventricular stroke volume via Starling's law.
7 Very quickly, a new steady state will be reached when left atrial pressure has risen sufficiently to make left ventricular stroke volume exactly equal to the increased right ventricular stroke volume.

The major conclusion here is that left atrial pressure will automatically change in the correct direction to match left ventricular stroke volume to the current right ventricular stroke volume. Consequently, it is usually an acceptable simplification to say that central venous pressure affects cardiac output as if the heart consisted only of a single pump.

Note that in Fig. 9-4, cardiac output and venous return are equal (at 5 liters/min) *only* when the central venous pressure is 2 mmHg. If central venous pressure were to decrease to 0 mmHg for any reason, cardiac output would fall (to 2 liters/min) and venous return would increase (to 7 liters/min). With a venous return of 7 liters/min and a cardiac output of 2 liters/min, the volume of the central venous pool would necessarily be increasing and this would produce a progressively increasing central venous pressure. In this manner, central venous pressure would return to the original level (2 mmHg) in a very short time. In contrast, if central venous pressure were to increase from 2 to 4 mmHg for any reason, venous return would decrease (to 3 liters/min) and cardiac output would increase (to 7 liters/min). This would quickly decrease the volume of blood in the central venous pool, and the central venous pressure would soon fall back to the original level. The cardiovascular system automatically adjusts to operate at the point where the cardiac output and venous return curves intersect. *Central venous pressure is always inherently driven to the equilibrium value that makes cardiac output and venous return equal. Cardiac output (and venous return) always stabilizes at the level where the cardiac output and venous return curves intersect.*

In order to fulfill its homeostatic role in the body, the cardiovascular system must be able to alter its cardiac output. Recall from Chap. 4 that cardiac output is affected by more than just cardiac filling pressure and that at any moment the heart may be operating on any one of a number of cardiac output curves, depending on the existing level of cardiac sympathetic tone (Fig. 4-10). The family of possible cardiac output curves may be plotted along with the family of possible venous return curves, as shown in Fig. 9-5. At a particular moment, the existing influences on the heart dictate the particular cardiac output curve on which it is working, and similarly, the existing influences on peripheral venous pressure dictate the particular venous return curve that applies. Thus, the influences on the heart and on the peripheral vasculature determine where the cardiac output and venous return curves intersect and thus what the central venous pressure and cardiac output (and venous return) are at equilibrium. In the intact cardiovascular

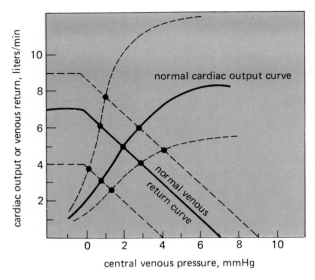

Figure 9-5   Families of cardiac output and venous return curves. Intersection points indicate equilibrium values for cardiac output, venous return, and central venous pressure.

system, cardiac output can rise only when the point of intersection of the cardiac output and venous return curves is raised. *All changes in cardiac output are caused by a shift in the cardiac output curve, a shift in the venous return curve, or both.*

The cardiac output and venous return curves are useful for understanding the complex interactions that occur in the intact cardiovascular system. With the help of Fig. 9-6, let us consider, for example, what happens to the cardiovascular system when there is a significant loss of blood (hemorrhage). We assume that before the hemorrhage, sympathetic tone to the heart and peripheral vessels is normal, as is the blood volume. Therefore cardiac output is related to central venous pressure as indicated by the "normal" cardiac output curve in Fig. 9-6. In addition, venous return is determined by central venous pressure as indicated by the "normal" venous return curve shown. The normal cardiac output and venous return curves intersect at point A, so cardiac output is 5 liters/min and central venous pressure is 2 mmHg. When blood volume decreases due to hemorrhage, the peripheral venous pressure falls and the venous return curve is shifted to the left. In the absence of any cardiovascular responses, the cardiovascular system must switch its operation to point B because this is now the point at which the cardiac output curve and the new venous return curve intersect. At the moment of blood loss, the venous return curve is shifted and venous return falls below cardiac output at the central venous pressure of 2 mmHg. This is what leads to the fall in the central venous pool volume and pressure that causes the shift in operation from point A to point B. Note by comparing points A and B in Fig. 9-6

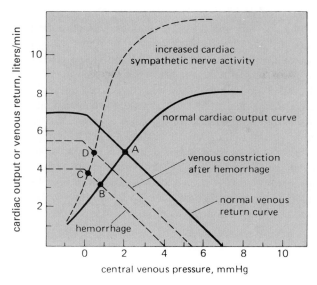

Figure 9-6   Cardiovascular adjustments to hemorrhage.

that blood loss itself lowers cardiac output *and* central venous pressure by shifting the venous return curve.

Subnormal cardiac output evokes a number of cardiovascular compensatory mechanisms in order to bring cardiac output back to more normal levels. One of these compensatory mechanisms is an increase in the activity of cardiac sympathetic nerves which shifts the heart's operation to a cardiac function curve that is higher than normal. The effect of increasing cardiac sympathetic activity is illustrated by a shift in cardiovascular operation from point B to point C. In itself, the increased cardiac sympathetic nerve activity increases cardiac output (from 3 to 4 liters/min) but causes a further decrease in central venous pressure. This drop in central venous pressure occurs because points B and C lie on the same venous return curve. *Cardiac* sympathetic nerves do not affect the venous return curve.[2]

An additional compensatory mechanism evoked by blood loss is increased activity of the sympathetic nerves leading to veins. Recall that this raises peripheral venous pressure and causes a rightward shift of the venous return curve. Therefore, increased sympathetic activity to veins tends to shift the venous return curve, originally lowered by blood loss, back toward normal. As a consequence of the increased peripheral venous tone and the shift to a more normal venous return curve, the cardiovascular operation shifts from point C to point D in Fig. 9-6. Thus peripheral venous constriction increases cardiac output by

---

[2]   Venous return is higher at point C than at point B, but the venous return curve has not shifted.

increasing central venous pressure and moving the heart's operation upward along a fixed cardiac function curve. It must be pointed out that separating the response to hemorrhage into distinct, progressive steps (i.e., A to B to C to D) is only a conceptualization for appreciating the individual effects of the different processes involved. In reality, the reflex venous and cardiac responses occur simultaneously and so quickly that they will easily keep up with the blood loss as it occurs. Thus, the actual course of a patient's net response to hemorrhage would follow nearly a straight line from point A to point D.

In summary, point D illustrates that normal cardiac output can be sustained in the face of blood loss by the combined effect of peripheral and cardiac adjustments. Hemorrhage is only one of an almost infinite variety of disturbances to the cardiovascular system. Plots such as those shown in Fig. 9-6 are very useful for understanding the many disturbances to the cardiovascular system and the ways in which they may be compensated.

CLINICAL IMPLICATIONS
OF ABNORMAL CENTRAL VENOUS PRESSURES

Although, in the clinical situation, we have no way to actually determine either cardiac output or venous return curves, we can obtain important information about the patient's circulatory status from measures of central venous pressure. As we have just shown, both venous return and cardiac output interact to determine the specific central venous pressure at any given time. Furthermore, circulatory filling (i.e., blood volume) is one of the primary determinants of the position of the venous return curve. Therefore, if a patient has *abnormally high* central venous pressure, either cardiac output is significantly depressed or blood volume is significantly elevated (or both). In contrast, if the patient has *abnormally low* central venous pressure, either cardiac output is significantly increased or blood volume is significantly low (or both).[3]

Rough estimates of central venous pressure can be obtained quite easily by observing the external jugular veins. Since the force of gravity tends to keep veins in the head and neck collapsed when an individual is in an upright position, there should be no distention (or retrograde pulsations from atrial contractions) observed in these neck veins. Conversely, when an individual is fully recumbent, the neck veins should be full and pulsations easily detected. Since normal central venous pressure is about 2 mmHg (7 cmH$_2$O), the veins will be filled about 7 cm above the right atrium. If a normal individual is placed in a semirecumbent position so that the external jugular veins are positioned at 7 cm above the right atrium, the point between the collapsed venous segment and the filled segment can be visualized. Abnormally high central venous pressures will

---

[3]   A normal central venous pressure, however, does not necessarily mean that cardiac output and blood volume are normal. As can be seen by inspection of the curves in Fig. 9-5, simultaneous upward or downward shifts of both the venous return and cardiac output curves can occur with little or no change in central venous pressure.

be associated with neck vein distention at a higher level (perhaps even when the patient is upright).

Because of its diagnostic value in critical care situations, central venous pressure is often monitored continuously via a catheter that is inserted in a peripheral vein and advanced centrally until its tip is in the central venous pool (i.e., near or in the right atrium). In some situations, it is desirable to assess *left atrial* pressure, which is the filling pressure for the left side of the heart. This is commonly done with a specialized flow-directed venous catheter that utilizes a small inflatable balloon at its tip to drag it with the blood flow through the right ventricle and pulmonic valve into the pulmonary artery. The balloon is then deflated and the cannula is advanced further until it wedges into a terminal branch of the pulmonary vasculature. The "pulmonary wedge pressure" recorded at this junction provides a useful estimate of left atrial pressure.

Study Questions: 42 to 44

10

REGULATION OF ARTERIAL PRESSURE

OBJECTIVES

The student understands the mechanisms involved in the short-term regulation of arterial pressure:

1 Identifies the sensory receptors, afferent pathways, central integrating centers, efferent pathways, and effector organs that participate in the arterial baroreceptor reflex.
2 States the location of the arterial baroreceptors and describes their operation.
3 Describes how changes in the neural activity in the pressor and depressor regions of the medullary cardiovascular centers influence the activity of the sympathetic and parasympathetic preganglionic fibers.
4 Describes how changes in the afferent input from arterial baroreceptors influence the neural activities in the pressor and depressor regions of the medullary cardiovascular centers.
5 Describes how the sympathetic and parasympathetic outputs from the medullary cardiovascular centers change in response to changes in arterial pressure.
6 Diagrams the chain of events that are initiated by the arterial baroreceptor reflex to compensate for a change in arterial pressure.
7 Describes how inputs to the medullary cardiovascular centers from cardiopulmonary baroreceptors, arterial and central chemoreceptors, receptors in skeletal muscle, the cerebral cortex, and the hypothalamus influence sympathetic activity, parasympathetic activity, and mean arterial pressure.
8 Describes and indicates the mechanisms involved in the Bezold-Jarisch reflex, the cerebral ischemic response, the Cushing reflex, the alerting reaction, blushing, vasovagal syncope, the dive reflex, and the cardiovascular responses to emotion and pain.
9 Graphs the relationships between mean arterial pressure and sympathetic nerve activity that describe the overall operation of (1) the heart

and peripheral vessels and (2) the arterial baroreceptors plus the medullary cardiovascular centers. Uses the graphs to do the following:

a State what determines the normal mean arterial pressure and the normal level of sympathetic nerve activity.

b Indicate how the relationship between sympathetic nerve activity and arterial pressure is shifted by a disturbance on the heart or vessels and how this alters the equilibrium within the arterial baroreceptor reflex control system.

c Indicate how the relationship between mean arterial pressure and sympathetic nerve activity is altered by inputs to the medullary cardiovascular centers not from arterial baroreceptors and how these shift the equilibrium within the arterial baroreceptor reflex control system.

The student understands the mechanisms involved in the long-term regulation of arterial pressure:

10 Describes baroreceptor adaptation.

11 Describes the influence of changes in body fluid volume on arterial pressure.

12 Indicates the mechanisms whereby altered arterial pressure alters glomerular filtration rate and renal tubular function to influence urine output.

13 Describes how mean arterial pressure is adjusted in the long term to that which causes fluid output rate to equal fluid intake rate.

Appropriate systemic arterial pressure is perhaps the single most important requirement for proper operation of the cardiovascular system. Without sufficient arterial pressure, the brain and the heart do not receive adequate blood flow no matter what adjustments are made in their vascular resistance by local control mechanisms. In contrast, unnecessary demands are placed on the heart by excessive arterial pressure. In this chapter we will discuss the elaborate mechanisms that have evolved for regulating this critical cardiovascular variable.

Arterial pressure is continuously monitored by various sensors located within the body. Whenever arterial pressure varies from normal, multiple reflex responses are initiated which cause the adjustments in cardiac output and total peripheral resistance needed to return arterial pressure to its normal value. In the short term (seconds), these adjustments are brought about by changes in the activity of the autonomic nerves leading to the heart and peripheral vessels. In the long term (minutes to days), other mechanisms such as changes in cardiac output brought about by changes in blood volume play an increasingly important role in the control of arterial pressure. We will first consider nervous reflexes that control arterial pressure in the short term and how these cardiovascular reflexes may be modulated in special instances by neural influences from outside the major cardiovascular control area in the central nervous system.

SHORT-TERM REGULATION OF ARTERIAL PRESSURE
Arterial Baroreceptor Reflex

The arterial *baroreceptor reflex* is the most important mechanism providing short-term regulation of arterial pressure. Recall that the usual components of a reflex pathway include sensory receptors, afferent pathways, integrating centers in the central nervous system, efferent pathways, and effector organs. As shown in Fig. 10-1, the efferent pathways of the arterial baroreceptor reflex are the cardiovascular sympathetic and cardiac parasympathetic nerves. The effector organs are the heart and peripheral blood vessels. We have not yet considered the sensory elements, the afferent pathways, or the integrating centers in the brain stem that make the reflex complete.

Efferent Pathways   In previous chapters, we have discussed the many actions of the sympathetic and parasympathetic nerves leading to the heart and blood vessels. For both systems, *postganglionic fibers,* whose cell bodies are in ganglia outside the central nervous system, form the terminal link to the heart and vessels. The influences of these postganglionic fibers on key cardiovascular variables are summarized in Fig. 10-1.

The activity of the terminal postganglionic fibers of the autonomic nervous system is determined by the activity of *preganglionic fibers* whose cell bodies lie within the central nervous system. In the sympathetic pathways, the cell bodies of the preganglionic fibers are located within the spinal cord. These preganglionic neurons have spontaneous activity that is modulated by excitatory and inhibitory inputs which arise from centers in the brain stem and descend in distinct *excitatory* and *inhibitory* spinal pathways. In the parasympathetic system, the cell bodies of the preganglionic fibers are located within the brain stem. Their spontaneous activity is modulated by inputs from adjacent centers in the brain stem.

Afferent Pathways   Sensory receptors, called *arterial baroreceptors,* are found in abundance in the walls of the aorta and carotid arteries. Major concentrations of these receptors are found near the arch of the aorta (the *aortic baroreceptors*) and at the bifurcation of the common carotid artery into the internal and external carotid arteries on either side of the neck (the *carotid sinus baroreceptors*). The receptors themselves are mechanoreceptors that sense arterial pressure indirectly from the degree of stretch of the elastic arterial walls.[1] In general, *increased stretch causes an increased action potential generation rate by the arterial baroreceptors.* Baroreceptors actually sense not only absolute stretch but also the rate of change of stretch. For this reason, both the mean arterial pressure and arterial pulse pressure affect baroreceptor firing rate as indicated in Fig. 10-2.

---

[1]   Baroreceptor discharge rate can be enhanced by mechanical manipulation of the arterial walls. For example, the carotid sinus baroreceptor firing rate can be increased by massaging the neck over the carotid sinus area.

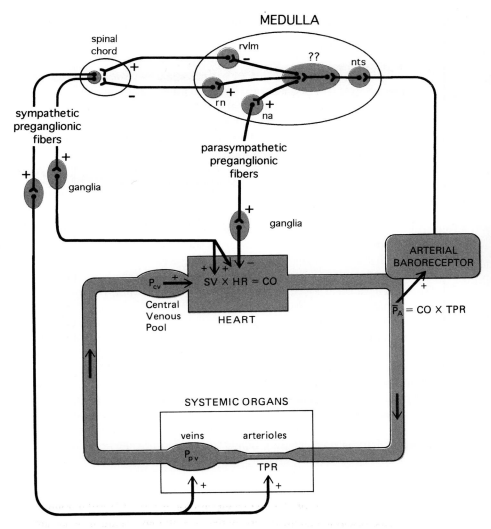

Figure 10-1 Components of the arterial baroreceptor reflex pathway. nts, nucleus tractus soli-tarius; rvlm, rostral ventrolateral medullary group; rn, raphé nucleus; na, nucleus ambiguus; ??, incompletely mapped integration pathways that may also involve structures outside the medulla.

The dashed curve in Fig. 10-2 shows how baroreceptor firing rate is affected by different levels of a steady arterial pressure. The solid curve in Fig. 10-2 indicates how baroreceptor firing rate is affected by the mean value of a pulsatile arterial pressure. Note that the presence of pulsations (which, of course, are normal) increases the baroreceptor firing rate at any given level of mean arterial

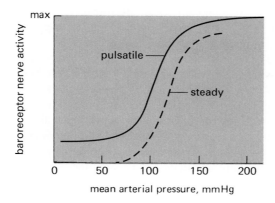

Figure 10-2   Effect of mean arterial pressure on baroreceptor nerve activity.

pressure. Note also that changes in mean arterial pressure near the normal value of 100 mmHg produce the largest changes in baroreceptor discharge rate.

If arterial pressure remains elevated over a period of several days for some reason, the arterial baroreceptor firing rate will gradually return toward normal. Thus arterial baroreceptors are said to *adapt* to long-term changes in arterial pressure. For this reason, the arterial baroreceptor reflex cannot serve as a mechanism for the long-range regulation of arterial pressure.

Action potentials generated by the carotid sinus baroreceptors travel through the carotid sinus nerves (Hering's nerves), which join with the glossopharyngeal nerves (ninth cranial nerves) before entering the central nervous system. Afferent fibers from the aortic baroreceptors run to the central nervous system in the vagus nerves (tenth cranial nerves). (The vagus nerves contain both afferent and efferent fibers, including, for example, the parasympathetic efferent fibers to the heart.)

Central Integration   Much of the central integration involved in reflex regulation of the cardiovascular system occurs in the medulla oblongata in what are traditionally referred to as the *medullary cardiovascular centers*. The neural interconnections between the diffuse structures in this area are complex and not completely mapped. Moreover, these structures appear to serve multiple functions including respiratory control, for example. What is known with a fair degree of certainty is where the cardiovascular afferent and efferent pathways enter and leave the medulla. For example, as indicated in Fig. 10-1, the afferent sensory information from the arterial baroreceptors enters the medullary *nucleus tractus solitarius* where it is relayed via polysynaptic pathways to other structures in the medulla (and higher brain centers, such as hypothalamus, as well). The cell bodies of the efferent vagal parasympathetic cardiac nerves are located primarily in the medullary *nucleus ambiguus*, which has also been called the "cardioinhibitory center." The sympathetic autonomic efferent information leaves the medulla predominantly from the *rostral ventrolateral medulla* group of neurons (via an excitatory spinal pathway) or the *raphé nucleus* (via an inhibitory spinal pathway). The intermediate processes involved in the actual integration of the sensory information into appropriate sympathetic and parasympathetic responses are not well understood at present. While much of this integration takes place within the medulla, higher centers such as the hypothalamus are probably involved as well. For our purposes, knowing details of the integration process are not as important as appreciating the overall effects that changes in arterial baroreceptor activity have on the activities of parasympathetic and sympathetic cardiovascular nerves.

Several functionally important points about the central control of the autonomic cardiovascular nerves are illustrated in Fig. 10-1. The major external influence on the cardiovascular centers comes from the arterial baroreceptors. Since the arterial baroreceptors are active at normal arterial pressures, they supply a tonic input to the central integration centers. As indicated in Fig. 10-1, the integration process is such that increased input from the arterial baroreceptors tends to simultaneously: (1) inhibit the activity of the spinal sympathetic excitatory tract, (2) stimulate the activity of the spinal sympathetic inhibitory tract, and (3) stimulate the activity of parasympathetic preganglionic nerves. Thus, an increase in the arterial baroreceptor discharge rate (caused by increased arterial pressure) causes a decrease in the tonic activity of cardiovascular sympathetic nerves and a simultaneous increase in the tonic activity of cardiac parasympathetic nerves. Conversely, decreased arterial pressure causes increased sympathetic and decreased parasympathetic activity.

Operation of the Arterial Baroreceptor Reflex   The arterial baroreceptor reflex is a continuously operating control system that automatically makes adjustments which prevent disturbances on the heart and vessels from causing large changes in mean arterial pressure. The arterial baroreceptor reflex mechanism acts to regulate arterial pressure in a *negative feedback* manner, which is analogous in many ways to the manner in which a thermostatically controlled home heating system operates to regulate inside temperature despite disturbances such as changes in the weather or open windows.[2]

Figure 10-3 shows many events in the arterial baroreceptor reflex pathway that occur in response to the stimulus of decreased mean arterial pressure. We have already discussed all of the events shown in Fig. 10-3, and each should be carefully examined (and reviewed if necessary) at this point because a great

[2]   In this analogy, arterial pressure is likened to temperature; the heart is the generator of pressure as the furnace is the generator of heat; dilated arterioles dissipate arterial pressure like open windows lose heat; the arterial baroreceptors monitor arterial pressure as the sensor of a thermostat monitors temperature; and the electronics of the thermostat control the furnace as the medullary cardiovascular centers regulate the operation of the heart. (Since home thermostats do not usually also regulate the operation of windows, there is no analogy to the reflex medullary control of arterioles. Also, there is no real equivalent of veins in a home heating system.) The pressure that the arterial baroreflex strives to maintain is analogous to the temperature setting on the thermostat dial.

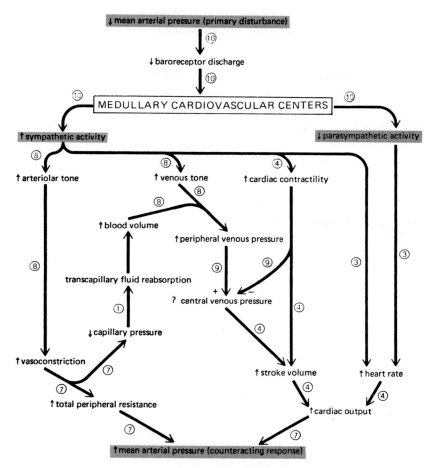

Figure 10-3 Immediate cardiovascular adjustments caused by a decrease in arterial blood pressure. Circled numbers indicate the chapter in which each interaction is discussed.

many of the interactions that are essential to understanding cardiovascular physiology are summarized in this figure.

Note in Fig. 10-3 that the overall response of the arterial baroreceptor reflex to the stimulus of decreased mean arterial pressure is increased mean arterial pressure (i.e., the response tends to remove the stimulus). A stimulus of increased mean arterial pressure would elicit events exactly opposite to those shown in Fig. 10-3 and produce the response of decreased mean arterial pressure; again, the response tends to remove the stimulus. Again, the arterial baroreceptor reflex is a negative feedback mechanism that operates automatically to resist changes in mean arterial pressure. The homeostatic benefits of the reflex action should be apparent.

One should recall that nervous control of vessels is more important in some areas such as the kidney, the skin, and the splanchnic organs than in the brain and heart muscle. Thus the reflex response to a fall in arterial pressure may, for example, include a significant increase in renal vascular resistance and a decrease in renal blood flow without changing the cerebral vascular resistance or blood flow. The peripheral vascular adjustments associated with the arterial baroreceptor reflex take place primarily in organs with strong sympathetic vascular control.

Other Cardiovascular Reflexes and Responses

Seemingly in spite of the arterial baroreceptor reflex mechanism, large and rapid changes in mean arterial pressure occur in certain physiological and pathological situations. These reactions are caused by influences on the medullary cardiovascular centers *other* than those from the arterial baroreceptors. As outlined in the following sections, these inputs on the medullary cardiovascular centers arise from many types of peripheral and central receptors as well as from "higher centers" in the central nervous system such as the hypothalamus and the cortex.

We made the analogy earlier that the arterial baroreceptor reflex operates to control arterial pressure somewhat as a home heating system acts to control inside temperature. Such a system automatically acts to counteract changes in temperature caused by such things as an open window.[3] It does not however resist changes in temperature caused by someone's resetting of the thermostat dial — in fact, the basic temperature regulating mechanisms cooperate wholeheartedly in adjusting the temperature to the new desired value. The temperature setting on a home thermostat's dial has a useful conceptual analogy in cardiovascular physiology often referred to as the *"set point"* for arterial pressure. *The many influences that we are about to discuss all influence arterial pressure as if they changed the arterial baroreceptor reflex's set point for pressure regulation.* Consequently, the arterial baroreceptor reflex does not resist these pressure disturbances but actually assists in producing them.

Reflexes from Receptors in Heart and Lungs   A host of mechanoreceptors and chemoreceptors that can elicit reflex cardiovascular responses have been identified in the atria, ventricles, coronary vessels, and the lungs. The role of these *cardiopulmonary receptors* in the neurohumoral control of the cardiovascular system is, in most cases, incompletely understood, but evidence is accumulating that they may be involved significantly in many physiological and pathological states.

One general function that the cardiopulmonary receptors perform is sensing the pressure (or volume) in the atria and central venous pool. Increased central venous pressure and volume cause receptor activation by stretch which elicits a reflex decrease in sympathetic activity. Decreased central venous pressure pro-

---

[3]   In Minnesota, an open window is an obvious temperature lowering disturbance.

duces the opposite response. There is currently much debate over how such *cardiopulmonary baroreflexes* interact with the arterial baroreflexes in overall cardiovascular regulation. The traditional view is that the cardiopulmonary baroreceptors are most important in the renal mechanisms of fluid volume regulation (which will be discussed in a later section of this chapter), while the arterial baroreceptors have more influence on the moment-to-moment regulation of cardiac output, total peripheral resistance, and thus arterial pressure. As with most straightforward and attractive hypotheses, the evidence, as it has accumulated, does not support such a clear division of labor between the arterial baroreceptors and the cardiopulmonary baroreceptors. Whatever the details, it is clear that cardiopulmonary baroreflexes normally exert a tonic inhibitory influence on sympathetic activity and play an important, but not yet completely defined, role in normal cardiovascular regulation.

Certain other reflexes originating from receptors in the cardiopulmonary region have been described, which may be important in specific pathological situations. For example, the *Bezold-Jarisch reflex,* which involves marked bradycardia and hypotension, is elicited by application of strong stimuli to coronary vessel (or myocardial) chemoreceptors concentrated primarily in the posterior wall of the left ventricle. There is much clinical evidence that myocardial infarctions involving this region of the ventricle can elicit the Bezold-Jarisch reflex. (Far more commonly, myocardial infarct patients have *hypotension,* as would be expected from compromised myocardial function, and *tachycardia* as would be expected from an arterial baroreceptor response to hypotension.)

Chemoreceptor Reflexes   Low P_{O_2} and/or high P_{CO_2} levels in the arterial blood cause reflex increases in respiratory rate *and* mean arterial pressure. This appears to be a result of increased activity of *arterial chemoreceptors,* located in the carotid arteries and the arch of the aorta, and *central chemoreceptors,* located somewhere within the central nervous system. Chemoreceptors probably play little role in the normal regulation of arterial pressure since arterial blood P_{O_2} and P_{CO_2} are normally held very nearly constant by respiratory control mechanisms.

An extremely strong reaction called the *cerebral ischemic response* is triggered by inadequate brain blood flow (ischemia) and can produce a more intense sympathetic vasoconstriction and cardiac stimulation than is elicited by any other influence on the cardiovascular control centers. Presumably the cerebral ischemic response is initiated by chemoreceptors located within the central nervous system. If cerebral blood flow is severely inadequate for several minutes, the cerebral ischemic response wanes and is replaced by marked loss of sympathetic activity. Presumably this situation results when function of the nerve cells in the cardiovascular centers become directly depressed by the unfavorable chemical conditions in the cerebrospinal fluid.

Whenever intracranial pressure is increased—for example, by tumor growth or trauma-induced bleeding within the rigid cranium—there is a parallel rise in arterial pressure. This is called the *Cushing reflex.* It can cause mean arterial pressures of more than 200 mmHg in severe cases of intracranial pressure elevation. The obvious benefit of the Cushing reflex is that it prevents collapse of cranial vessels and thus preserves adequate brain blood flow in the face of large increases in intracranial pressure. The mechanisms responsible for the Cushing reflex are not known but could involve the central chemoreceptors.

Reflexes from Receptors in Exercising Skeletal Muscle   Reflex tachycardia and increased arterial pressure can be elicited by stimulation of certain afferent fibers from skeletal muscle. These pathways may be activated by chemoreceptors responding to muscle ischemia, which occurs with strong, sustained static (isometric) exercise. This input may contribute to the marked increase in blood pressure which accompanies such effort. It is uncertain as to what extent this reflex contributes to the cardiovascular responses to dynamic (rhythmic) muscle exercise.

The Dive Reflex   Aquatic animals respond to diving with a remarkable bradycardia and intense vasoconstriction in all systemic organs except the brain and heart. The response serves to allow prolonged submersion by limiting the rate of oxygen use and by directing blood flow to essential organs. A similar but less dramatic dive reflex can be elicited in humans by simply immersing the face in cold water. (Cold water enhances the response.) The response involves the unusual combination of bradycardia produced by enhanced cardiac parasympathetic activity and peripheral vasoconstriction caused by enhanced sympathetic activity which is a rare exception to the general rule that sympathetic and parasympathetic nerves are activated in reciprocal fashion. The dive reflex is sometimes used clinically (as is carotid massage) to activate cardiac parasympathetic nerves for the purpose of interrupting atrial tachyarrhythmias.

Cardiovascular Responses Associated with Emotion   Cardiovascular responses are frequently associated with certain states of emotion. These responses originate in the cerebral cortex and reach the medullary cardiovascular centers through corticohypothalamic pathways. The least complicated of these responses is the *blushing* that is often detectable in individuals with lightly pigmented skin during states of embarrassment. The blushing response involves a loss of sympathetic vasoconstrictor activity *only* to cutaneous vessels, and this produces the blushing by allowing engorgement of the cutaneous venous sinuses.

Excitement or a sense of danger often elicits a complex behavioral pattern called the *alerting reaction* (also called the "defense" or "fight or flight" response). The alerting reaction involves a host of responses such as pupillary dilation and increased skeletal muscle tenseness, which are generally appropriate preparations for some form of intense physical activity. The cardiovascular component of the alerting reaction is an increase in blood pressure caused by a general increase in cardiovascular sympathetic nervous activity and a decrease in cardiac parasympathetic activity. Centers in the *posterior hypothalamus* are presumed to be involved in the alerting reaction since many of the components of this multifaceted response can be experimentally reproduced by electrical stimulation of this area. The general cardiovascular effects are mediated via hypothalamic communications with the medullary cardiovascular centers.

Some individuals respond to situations of extreme stress by fainting, a situation referred to clinically as *vasovagal syncope*. The loss of consciousness is due to decreased cerebral blood flow, which is itself produced by a sudden dramatic loss of arterial blood pressure which, in turn, occurs as a result of a sudden loss of sympathetic tone and a simultaneous large increase in parasympathetic tone and decrease in heart rate. The influences on the medullary cardiovascular centers which produce vasovagal syncope appear to come from the cortex via depressor centers in the *anterior hypothalamus*. It has been suggested that vasovagal syncope is analogous to the "playing dead" response to peril utilized by some animals. Fortunately, unconsciousness (combined with becoming horizontal) seems to quickly remove this serious disturbance on the normal mechanisms of arterial pressure control in humans.

The extent to which cardiovascular variables, in particular blood pressure, are normally affected by emotional state is currently a topic of extreme interest and considerable research. As yet the answer is unclear. However, the therapeutic value of being able, for example, to learn to consciously reduce one's blood pressure would be incalculable.

Central Command   The term *central command* is used to imply an input from the cerebral cortex to lower brain centers during voluntary muscle exercise. The concept is that the same cortical drives that initiate somatomotor (skeletal muscle) activity also simultaneously initiate cardiovascular (and respiratory) adjustments appropriate to support that activity. In the absence of any other obvious causes, central command is at present the best explanation as to why both mean arterial pressure and respiration increase during voluntary exercise.

Reflex Responses to Pain   Pain can have either a positive or negative influence on arterial pressure. Generally, superficial or cutaneous pain causes a rise in blood pressure in a manner similar to that associated with the alerting response and perhaps over many of the same pathways. Deep pain from receptors in the viscera or joints, however, often causes a cardiovascular response similar to that which accompanies vasovagal syncope, i.e., decreased sympathetic tone, increased parasympathetic tone, and a serious decrease in blood pressure. This response may contribute to the state of shock that often accompanies crushing injuries and/or joint displacement.

Temperature Regulation Reflexes   Certain special cardiovascular reflexes that involve the control of skin blood flow have evolved as part of the body temperature regulation mechanisms. Temperature regulation responses are controlled primarily by the hypothalamus, which can operate through the cardiovascular centers to discretely control the sympathetic activity to cutaneous vessels and thus skin blood flow. The sympathetic activity to cutaneous vessels is extremely responsive to changes in hypothalamic temperature. Measurable changes in cutaneous blood flow result from changes in hypothalamic temperature of tenths of a degree Celsius.

Cutaneous vessels are influenced by reflexes involved in both arterial pressure regulation and temperature regulation. When the appropriate cutaneous vascular responses for temperature regulation and pressure regulation are contradictory, as they are, for example, during strenuous exercise in a hot environment, then the temperature-regulating influences on cutaneous blood vessels usually prevail.

Summary   Most of the influences on the medullary cardiovascular centers that have been discussed in the preceding sections are summarized in Fig. 10-4. This figure is intended first to reemphasize that the arterial baroreceptors normally supply the major input to the medullary centers. The arterial baroreceptor input is shown as inhibitory because an increase in arterial baroreceptor firing rate results in a decrease in sympathetic output. (Decreased sympathetic output should be taken to imply also a simultaneous increase in parasympathetic output which is not shown.) As indicated in Fig. 10-4, the nonarterial baroreceptor influences on the medullary cardiovascular centers fall into two categories: (1) those that *increase* arterial pressure by raising the set point for the arterial baroreceptor re-

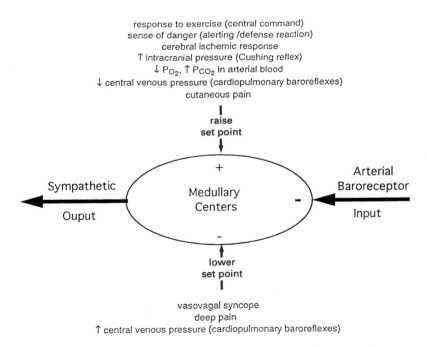

Figure 10-4 Summary of the factors that influence the set point of the arterial baroreceptor reflex.

flex and thus causing an increase in sympathetic activity, and (2) those that *decrease* arterial pressure by lowering the set point for the arterial baroreceptor reflex and thus causing a decrease in sympathetic activity. Note that certain responses which we have discussed are not included in Fig. 10-4. The complex combination of stimuli involved in the dive reflex cause simultaneous sympathetic and parasympathetic activation and cannot be simply classified as either pressure raising or pressure lowering. Also, stimuli which discretely affect cutaneous vessels but not general cardiovascular sympathetic and parasympathetic activity have not been included in Fig. 10-4.

The nonarterial baroreceptor influences shown in Fig. 10-4 may be viewed as disturbances on the cardiovascular system that act on the medullary cardiovascular centers. These disturbances cause sympathetic activity and arterial pressure to change in the *same direction*. Recall from the discussion of the arterial baroreceptor reflex that cardiovascular disturbances that act on the heart or vessels (such as blood loss or heart failure) produce *reciprocal* changes in arterial pressure and sympathetic activity.

Equilibrium in the Arterial Baroreceptor System

There are instances when it would appear that the arterial baroreceptor reflex is not working. For example, both arterial pressure and heart rate increase during exercise (as will be discussed fully in the next chapter). Would not one expect the baroreceptor reflex to decrease heart rate in response to increased arterial pressure? The material presented in the following section is designed to help the student understand such apparent inconsistencies.

The complete arterial baroreceptor reflex pathway is a control system made up of two distinct portions as shown in Fig. 10-5: (1) an *effector portion,* including the heart and peripheral blood vessels, and (2) a *neural portion* which includes the arterial baroreceptors, their afferent nerve fibers, the medullary cardiovascular centers, and the efferent sympathetic and parasympathetic fibers. Mean arterial pressure is the *output* of the effector portion and simultaneously the *input* to the neural portion. Similarly, the activity of the sympathetic (and parasympathetic)[4] cardiovascular nerves is the *output* of the neural portion of the arterial baroreceptor control system and, at the same time, the *input* to the effector portion.

In Chaps. 3 to 10 we discussed a host of reasons why mean arterial pressure *increases* when the heart and peripheral vessels receive *increased* sympathetic nerve activity. All this information is summarized by the curve shown in the lower graph of Fig. 10-5, which describes the effector portion of the arterial baroreceptor system alone. We have also discussed in this chapter how *increased* mean arterial pressure acts through the arterial baroreceptors and medullary

---

[4]   For convenience, we will omit continual reference to parasympathetic nerve activity in the following discussion. Throughout, however, an indicated change in sympathetic nerve activity should also be taken to imply a reciprocal change in the activity of the cardiac parasympathetic nerves unless otherwise noted.

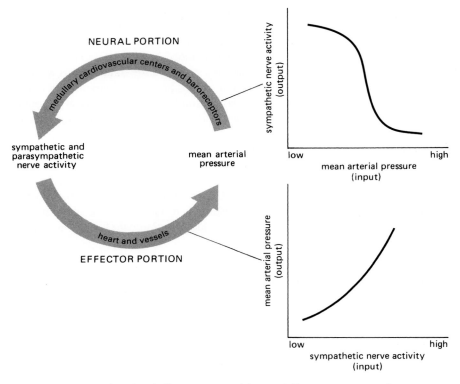

Figure 10-5   Neural and effector portions of the arterial baroreceptor control system.

cardiovascular centers to *decrease* the sympathetic activity. This information is summarized by the curve shown in the upper graph of Fig. 10-5, which describes the neural portion of the arterial baroreceptor system *alone*.

When the arterial baroreceptor system is intact and operating as a closed loop, the effector portion and neural portion retain their individual rules of operation as described by the individual function curves. Yet in the closed loop the two portions of the system must interact until they come into equilibrium with each other at some mutually compatible combination of mean arterial pressure and sympathetic activity. Equilibrium values of mean arterial pressure and sympathetic nerve activity can be determined by reversing the axes of the neural function curve and by plotting it together with the effector function curve on the same graph (as in Fig. 10-6A) and identified by the point of intersection of these two curves.

Whenever there is any outside disturbance on the cardiovascular system, the equilibrium point of the arterial baroreceptor system shifts. This happens because *all* cardiovascular disturbances cause a shift in one or the other of the two curves in Fig. 10-6A. For example, Fig. 10-6B shows how the equilibrium for the

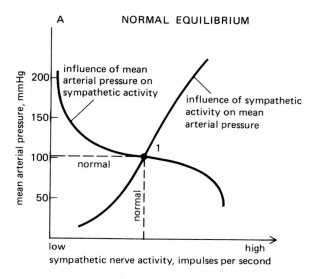

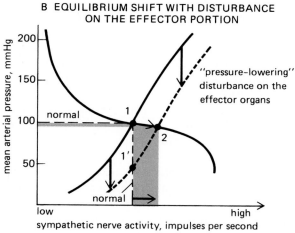

Figure 10-6 Operation of the arterial baroreceptor control system. A. Normal equilibrium. B. Equilibrium shift with disturbance on the effector portion.

arterial baroreceptor system is shifted by a cardiovascular disturbance that lowers the operating curve of the effector portion. The disturbance in this case could be anything that reduces the arterial pressure produced by the heart and vessels *at each given level of sympathetic activity.* Blood loss, for example, is such a disturbance because it lowers central venous pressure and through the Frank-Starling law, lowers cardiac output and thus mean arterial pressure at any given level of cardiac sympathetic nerve activity. Metabolic vasodilation of arterioles in exercising skeletal muscle is another example of a pressure-lowering disturbance on the effector portion of the system because it lowers the total peripheral resistance and thus the arterial pressure that the heart and vessels produce at any given level of sympathetic nerve activity.

As shown by point 2 in Fig. 10-6B, any pressure-lowering disturbance on the heart or vessels causes a new equilibrium to be reached within the baroreceptor system at a slightly lower than normal mean arterial pressure and a higher than normal sympathetic activity level. Note that the point 1' in Fig. 10-6B indicates how far the mean arterial pressure would have fallen as a consequence of the disturbance had not the sympathetic activity been automatically increased above normal by the arterial baroreceptor system.

As indicated previously in this chapter, many disturbances act on the neural portion of the arterial baroreceptor system rather than directly on the heart or vessels. These disturbances shift the equilibrium within the cardiovascular system because they alter the operating curve of the neural portion of the system. For example, the influences listed in Fig. 10-4 that raise the set point shift the operating curve for the neural portion of the arterial baroreceptor system to the right as shown in Fig. 10-7A because they increase the level of sympathetic output from the medullary cardiovascular centers *at each and every level of arterial pressure* (i.e., at each and every level of input from the arterial baroreceptors). For example, a sense of danger will cause the components of the arterial baroreceptor system to reach equilibrium at a higher than normal arterial pressure and a higher than normal sympathetic activity as shown in Fig. 10-7A. Conversely, but not shown in Fig. 10-7, any of the set-point lowering influences listed in Fig. 10-4 acting on the medullary cardiovascular centers will shift the operating curve for the neural portion of the arterial baroreceptor system to the left and a new equilibrium will be reached at lower than normal arterial pressure and sympathetic activity.

Many physiological and pathological situations involve simultaneous disturbances on both the neural and effector portions of the arterial baroreceptor system. Figure 10-7B illustrates this type of situation. The set-point-increasing disturbance on the neural portion of the system alone causes the equilibrium to shift from point 1 to point 2. Superimposing a pressure-lowering disturbance on the heart or vessels further shifts the equilibrium from point 2 to point 3. Note that, although the response to the pressure-lowering disturbance in Fig. 10-7B (point 2 to point 3) starts from a higher than normal arterial pressure, it is essentially identical to that which occurs in the absence of a set-point-increasing influence on the cardiovascular center (see Fig. 10-6B). Thus, the response is an attempt to prevent the arterial pressure from falling below that at point 2. The overall implication is that any of the set-point-increasing influences on the medullary cardiovascular centers listed in Fig. 10-4 cause the arterial baroreceptor system to regulate arterial pressure to a higher than normal value. Conversely, the set-point-lowering influences on the medullary cardiovascular centers listed in Fig. 10-4 would cause the arterial baroreceptor system to regulate arterial pressure to a lower than normal value.

In the next chapters we will discuss many situations which involve a higher than normal sympathetic activity at a time when arterial pressure is itself higher than normal. It should be noted that higher than normal sympathetic activity and higher than normal arterial pressure can exist together only when there is a set-point-raising influence on the *neural* portion of the arterial baroreceptor system.

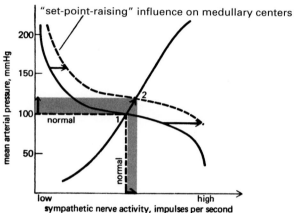

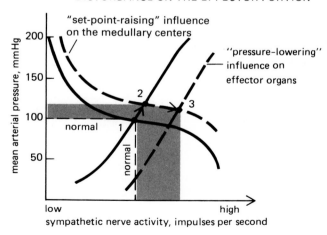

Figure 10-7 Effect of neural influences on the arterial baroreceptor control system. *A.* Equilibrium shift with disturbance on the neural portion. *B.* Equilibrium shift with disturbances on both neural and effector portions.

LONG-TERM REGULATION OF ARTERIAL PRESSURE

Fluid Balance and Arterial Pressure

We have already considered several key factors in the long-term regulation of arterial blood pressure. First is the fact that the baroreceptor reflex, however well it counteracts temporary disturbances in arterial pressure, cannot effectively regulate arterial pressure in the long term for the simple reason that the baroreceptor firing rate adapts to prolonged changes in arterial pressure.

The second pertinent fact is that circulating blood volume can influence arterial pressure because:

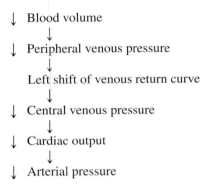

A fact we have yet to consider is that arterial pressure has a profound influence on urine output rate and thus affects total body fluid volume. Since blood volume is one of the components of the total body fluid, blood volume alterations accompany changes in total body fluid volume. The mechanisms are such that an *increase in arterial pressure* causes an increase in urine output rate and thus a *decrease in blood volume.* But, as outlined in the preceding sequence, decreased blood volume tends to lower arterial pressure. Thus, the complete sequence of events that are initiated by an increase in arterial pressure can be listed as follows:

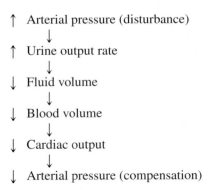

Note the negative feedback nature of this sequence of events: increased arterial pressure leads to fluid volume depletion, which tends to lower arterial

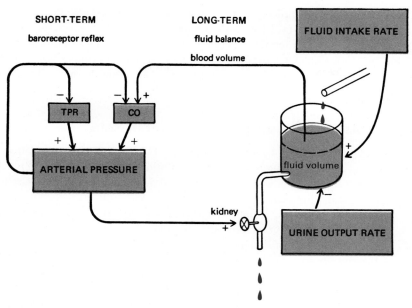

Figure 10-8 Mechanisms of short- and long-term regulation of arterial pressure. TPR, total peripheral resistance; CO, cardiac output.

pressure. Conversely, an initial disturbance of decreased arterial pressure would lead to fluid volume expansion, which would tend to increase arterial pressure. Because of negative feedback, these events constitute a *fluid volume mechanism* for regulating arterial pressure.

As indicated in Fig. 10-8, both the arterial baroreceptor reflex and this fluid volume mechanism are negative feedback loops that regulate arterial pressure. Whereas the arterial baroreceptor reflex is very quick to counteract disturbances in arterial pressure, hours or even days may be required before a change in urine output rate produces a significant accumulation or loss of total body fluid volume. Whatever this fluid volume mechanism lacks in speed, however, it more than makes up for in persistence. As long as there is *any* inequality between the fluid intake rate and the urine output rate, fluid volume is changing and this fluid volume mechanism has not completed its adjustment of arterial pressure. The fluid volume mechanism is in equilibrium only when the urine output rate exactly equals the fluid intake rate.[5] *In the long term, the arterial pressure can only be that which makes the urine output rate equal to the fluid intake rate.*

---

[5] In the present discussion, assume that fluid intake rate represents that in excess of the obligatory fluid losses which normally occur in the feces and by transpiration from the skin and structures in the respiratory tract. The processes that regulate voluntary fluid intake (thirst) are not well understood but seem to involve many of the same factors that influence urine output (e.g., blood volume and osmolality). Angiotensin II may be an important factor in the regulation of thirst.

The baroreceptor reflex is, of course, essential for counteracting rapid changes in arterial pressure. The fluid volume mechanism, however, determines the long-term level of arterial pressure because it slowly overwhelms all other influences. Through adaptation, the baroreceptor mechanism adjusts itself so that it operates to prevent acute changes in blood pressure from the prevailing long-term level as determined through fluid balance.

Effect of Arterial Pressure on Urine Output Rate

A key element in the fluid balance mechanism of arterial pressure regulation is the effect that arterial pressure has on the renal urine production rate. The mechanisms responsible for this will be only briefly described here with emphasis on their cardiovascular implications.

As indicated in Chap. 1, the kidneys play a major role in homeostasis by regulating the electrolyte composition of the plasma and thus the entire internal environment. One of the major plasma electrolytes regulated by the kidneys is the sodium ion. To regulate the electrolyte composition, a large fraction of the plasma fluid that flows into the kidneys is filtered across the *glomerular capillaries* so that it enters the *renal tubules*. The fluid that passes from the blood into the renal tubules is called the *glomerular filtrate,* and the rate at which this process occurs is called the *glomerular filtration rate.* Glomerular filtration is a transcapillary fluid movement whose rate is influenced by hydrostatic and oncotic pressures as indicated in Chap. 1. The primary cause of continual glomerular filtration is that glomerular capillary hydrostatic pressure is normally very high (≈ 70 mmHg). The glomerular filtration rate is decreased by factors that decrease glomerular capillary pressure, e.g., decreased arterial blood pressure or vasoconstriction of preglomerular renal arterioles.

Once fluid is filtered into the renal tubules, it either (1) is *reabsorbed* and reenters the cardiovascular system or (2) is passed along renal tubules and eventually *excreted* as urine. Thus urine production is the net result of glomerular filtration and renal tubular fluid reabsorption:

Urine output rate = glomerular filtration rate − renal fluid reabsorption rate

Actually, most of the reabsorption of fluid that has entered renal tubules as glomerular filtrate occurs because sodium is actively pumped out of the tubules by cells in the tubular wall. When sodium leaves the tubules, osmotic forces are produced that cause water to leave with it. Thus any factor that promotes renal tubular sodium reabsorption (sodium retention) tends to increase the renal fluid reabsorption rate and consequently decrease the urine output rate. The blood concentration of the hormone *aldosterone,* which is produced by the adrenal glands, is the primary regulator of the rate of sodium reabsorption by renal tubular cells. Adrenal release of aldosterone is, in turn, regulated largely by the circulating level of another hormone, *angiotensin II,* whose plasma concentration is determined by the plasma concentration of *renin,* an enzyme that is produced in the kidneys. Renin actually catalyzes the formation of an inactive decapeptide, *angiotensin I,* from *angiotensinogen,* a circulating precursor protein. Angiotensin I then gets quickly converted to angiotensin II (an octapeptide) by the action of *angiotensin converting enzyme (ACE)* which is located on the surface of endothelial cells. The combination of elements involved in this whole sequence of events is referred to as the *renin-angiotensin-aldosterone system.*

The rate of renin release by the kidneys appears to be influenced by several factors. An increase in the activity of renal sympathetic nerves causes a direct release of renin through a β_1-adrenergic mechanism. Also, renin release is triggered by factors associated with a lowered glomerular filtration rate. The activation of sympathetic vasoconstrictor nerves to renal arterioles thus indirectly causes renin release via lowered glomerular capillary hydrostatic pressure and glomerular filtration rate. The important fact to keep in mind, from a cardiovascular standpoint, is that anything that causes renin release causes a decrease in urine output rate because increased renin causes increased sodium (and therefore fluid) reabsorption from renal tubules.[6]

Urine output rate is also influenced by vasopressin (antidiuretic hormone, ADH) released from the posterior pituitary. Vasopressin regulates the permeability of certain portions of the kidney tubule is such a way that when the blood levels of the hormone are elevated, water is reabsorbed from the tubule and the kidney produces only small volumes of highly concentrated urine. The production of vasopressin in the hypothalamus and its release from the pituitary are stimulated by many factors including increased extracellular fluid osmolality, decreased input from cardiopulmonary baroreceptors, and decreased input from arterial baroreceptors. In the case of the latter two influences on vasopressin release, the overall result is to decrease urine output rate whenever arterial pressure and/or central blood volume are below normal.

Some major mechanisms that lead to decreased urine output rate are summarized in Fig. 10-9. Most importantly, this figure shows that urine output rate is linked to arterial pressure by many synergistic pathways. Because of this, modest changes in arterial pressure are associated with large changes in urine output rate.

The observed relation between arterial pressure and urine output for a normal person is shown in Fig. 10-10. Recall that, in the steady state, the urine output rate must always equal the fluid intake rate and that changes in fluid volume will automatically adjust arterial pressure until this is so. Thus a normal person

---

[6] Although the renin-angiotensin-aldosterone system is clearly the primary mechanism for the regulation of renal tubular sodium reabsorption, many believe that other factors are involved. A polypeptide natriuretic (salt-losing) factor has been identified in granules of cardiac atrial cells. Atrial distention causes the release of this *atrial natriuretic peptide* (ANP) into the blood. The possibility that the heart itself may serve as an endocrine organ in the regulation of body fluid volume is stimulating much research interest.

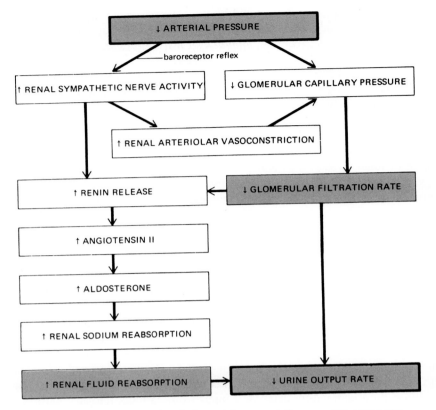

Figure 10-9   Mechanisms by which arterial pressure influences urine output rate.

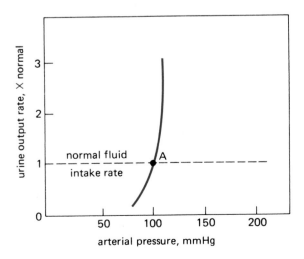

Figure 10-10   Effect of arterial pressure on urine output rate in a normal person.

with a normal fluid intake rate will have, as a long-term average, the arterial pressure associated with point A in Fig. 10-10. Because of the steepness of the curve shown in Fig. 10-10, even rather marked changes in fluid rate have rather minor influences on the arterial pressure of a normal individual.

Study Questions: 45 to 50

11

CARDIOVASCULAR RESPONSES TO PHYSIOLOGICAL STRESSES

OBJECTIVES

The student understands the general mechanisms involved in the cardiovascular responses to *any* given normal homeostatic disturbance on the intact cardiovascular system and can predict the resulting alterations in all important cardiovascular variables:

1 Identifies the primary disturbances that the situation places on the cardiovascular system.
2 Lists how the primary disturbances change the influence on the medullary cardiovascular centers from (1) arterial baroreceptors and (2) other sources.
3 States what changes will occur in sympathetic and parasympathetic nerve activities as a result of the altered influences on the medullary cardiovascular centers.
4 Indicates what immediate reflex changes will occur in heart rate, cardiac contractility, stroke volume, arteriolar tone, venous tone, peripheral venous pressure, central venous pressure, total peripheral resistance, resistance in any major organ, and blood flow through any major organ.
5 Predicts what the net effect of the primary and reflex influences on the cardiovascular variables listed in objective 4 will be on mean arterial pressure.
6 States whether mean arterial pressure and sympathetic nerve activity will settle above or below their normal values.
7 Predicts whether and states how cutaneous blood flow will be altered by temperature regulation reflexes.
8 Indicates whether and how transcapillary fluid movements will be involved in the overall cardiovascular response.
9 Indicates whether, why, how, and with what time course renal adjustments of fluid balance will participate in the response.
10 Predicts how each of the variables listed in objective 4 will be influenced by long-term adjustments in blood volume.

The student understands how respiratory activities influence the cardiovascular system:

11 Describes how the "respiratory pump" promotes venous return.
12 Identifies the primary disturbances on cardiovascular variables associated with normal respiratory activity.
13 Describes the reflex compensatory responses to respiratory activity.
14 Defines the causes of "normal sinus arrhythmia."
15 Lists the cardiovascular consequences of the Valsalva maneuver.

The student understands the specific processes associated with the homeostatic adjustments to the effects of gravity:

16 States how gravity influences arterial, venous, and capillary pressures at any height above or below the heart in a standing individual.
17 Describes and explains the changes in central venous pressure and the changes in transcapillary fluid balance and venous volume in the lower extremities caused by standing upright.
18 Describes the operation of the "skeletal muscle pump" and explains how it simultaneously promotes venous return and decreases capillary hydrostatic pressure in the muscle vascular beds.
19 Identifies the primary disturbances and compensatory responses evoked by acute changes in body position.
20 Describes the chronic effects of a gravity-free environment and compares these to those induced by long-term bed rest.

The student understands the specific processes associated with the homeostatic adjustments to exercise:

21 Identifies the primary disturbances and compensatory responses evoked by acute episodes of dynamic exercise.
22 Describes the conflict between pressure reflexes and temperature reflexes on cutaneous blood flow.
23 Indicates how the "skeletal muscle pump" and the "respiratory pump" contribute to cardiovascular adjustments during exercise.
24 Compares the cardiovascular responses to static exercise with those to dynamic exercise.
25 Lists the effects of chronic exercise and physical conditioning upon cardiovascular variables.

The student understands how age-dependent alterations in the cardiovascular system may influence responses to homeostatic disturbances.

26 Identifies age-dependent changes that occur in cardiovascular variables such as cardiac index, arterial pressure, and cardiac workload.
27 Describes age-dependent changes in the arterial baroreceptor reflex.
28 Distinguishes between age- and disease-dependent alterations that occur in cardiovascular function of the aged.

In this and the next chapter we will see how the basic principles of cardiovascular physiology, which have been discussed, apply to the intact cardiovascular system. A variety of situations that tend to disturb homeostasis will be presented. The key to understanding the cardiovascular adjustments in each situation is to recall that the arterial baroreceptor reflex and renal fluid balance mechanisms always act to blunt changes in arterial pressure. The overall result is that *adequate blood flow to the brain and the heart muscle is maintained in any circumstance.*

The cardiovascular alterations in each of the following examples are produced by the combined effects of (1) the primary, direct influences of the disturbance on the cardiovascular variables and (2) the reflex adjustments that are triggered by the primary disturbances. The general pattern of reflex adjustment is similar in all situations. Rather than trying to memorize the cardiovascular alterations that accompany each situation, the student should strive to understand each response in terms of the primary disturbances and reflex reactions involved. To aid in this process, a list of key cardiovascular variables and their determinants may be found in Appendix C.

An extensive list of study questions is supplied for Chaps. 11 and 12. These questions are intended to reinforce the student's understanding of complex cardiovascular responses and provide a review of basic cardiovascular principles.

EFFECT OF RESPIRATORY ACTIVITY

During a normal inspiration, intrathoracic pressure falls by about 7 mmHg as the diaphragm contracts and the chest wall expands and rises again by an equal amount during expiration. These periodic pressure fluctuations not only promote air movement into and out of the lungs but also are transmitted through the thin walls of the great veins in the thorax to influence venous return to the heart from the periphery. Because of the venous valves, venous return is increased more by inspiration than it is decreased by expiration. The net effect is that venous return from the periphery is generally facilitated by the periodic fluctuations in central venous pressure caused by respiration. This phenomenon is often referred to as the "respiratory pump."

Because of these changes in venous return, normal breathing is associated with transient cyclical changes in cardiac output and arterial pressure. Heart rate in normal individuals also fluctuates in syncrony with the respiratory rate. This is referred to as "normal sinus arrhythmia." Some of the major primary disturbances and compensatory responses involved in the cardiovascular effects of respiration are illustrated in Fig. 11-1, although the complete picture is much more complex than shown. Filling of the right side of the heart is transiently increased during inspiration and, by Starling's law, stroke volume and thus cardiac output are transiently increased. Since changes in output of the right side of the heart induce changes in output of the left side of the heart, the net effect of inspiration will be a transient increase in stroke volume and cardiac output from the left ventricle. This will lead to a transient increase in arterial pressure and a transient increase in firing of the arterial baroreceptors. In addition, because of the inspiration-induced decrease in intrathoracic pressure, the cardiopulmonary barore-

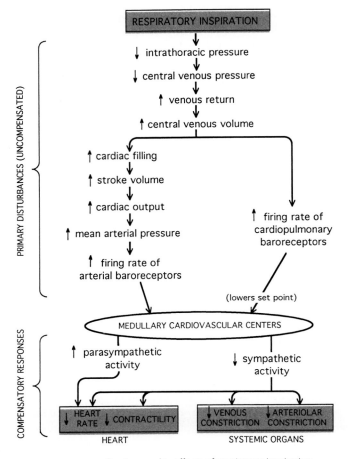

Figure 11-1   Cardiovascular effects of respiratory inspiration.

ceptors will be stretched and will increase their firing rate. These baroreceptor inputs will act on the medullary cardiovascular centers to produce reflex adjustments to lower arterial pressure: that is, increase cardiac parasympathetic nerve activity and decrease sympathetic nerve activity. Under normal resting conditions, the cyclic change in heart rate is the most apparent cardiovascular response to respiration.[1]

There are a number of instances when cardiovascular effects of respiratory

[1] Although the respiratory effects of right heart filling are emphasized in Fig. 11-1, respiration also directly affects left heart filling. However, the events are somewhat different because both the left atria and the whole of the pulmonary vascular system are affected by changes in intrathoracic pressure. There are also some time delays between changes in right heart filling and left ventricular stroke volume that are ignored in Fig. 11-1. The specific phase relationships between the respiratory cycle and the cardiovascular effects are influenced by respiratory rate and depth as well as the current average heart rate.

efforts are extremely important. In *exercise,* for example, a deep and rapid breathing rate contributes significantly to the venous return. *Yawning* is a complex event which includes a significant transient decrease in intrathoracic pressure that is effective in increasing venous return (especially when combined with stretching!). In contrast, *coughing* is associated with an *increase* in intrathoracic pressure and, if occurring as a "fit," can lead to such severe reductions in cardiac output as to cause fainting.

The cardiovascular consequences of changes in intrathoracic pressure are also important during the *Valsalva maneuver,* which is a forced expiration against a closed glottis. This maneuver is normally performed by individuals during defecation ("straining at stool"), or when attempting to lift a heavy object. (Similar conditions exist when forced expirations are made against a high output resistance, such as when blowing up one of those nasty little party balloons.) There are several phases in the cardiovascular reaction. At the initiation of the Valsalva maneuver, arterial pressure is abruptly elevated for several beats due to the intrathoracic pressure transmitted to the thoracic aorta. The sustained elevation in intrathoracic pressure leads to a fall in venous return and a fall in blood pressure, which evokes a reflex increase in heart rate and peripheral vaso-constriction. (During this period, the red face and distended peripheral veins are indicative of high peripheral venous pressures.) At the cessation of the maneuver, there is an abrupt fall in pressure for a couple of beats due to the reduction of intrathoracic pressure. Venous blood then moves rapidly into the central venous pool; stroke volume, cardiac output, and arterial pressure increase rapidly; and a reflex bradycardia occurs. The combination of an episode of high peripheral venous pressure followed by an episode of high arterial pressure and pulse pressure is particularly dangerous for people who are candidates for cerebral vascular accidents (strokes) because this combination may rupture a vessel.

EFFECT OF GRAVITY

Responses to Changes in Body Position

Because gravity has an effect on pressures within the cardiovascular system, significant cardiovascular readjustments accompany changes in body position. In the preceding chapters, the influence of gravity was ignored and pressure differences between various points in the systemic circulation were related only to flow and vascular resistance $(\Delta P = \dot{Q}R)$. As shown in Fig. 11-2, this is approximately true only for a recumbent individual. In a standing individual, additional cardiovascular pressure differences exist between the heart and regions that are not at heart level. This is most important in the lower legs and feet of a standing individual. As indicated in Fig. 11-2B, all intravascular pressures in the feet may be increased by 90 mmHg simply from the weight of the blood in the arteries and veins leading to and from the feet. Note by comparing Fig. 11-2A and B that standing upright does not in itself change the flow through the lower extremities, since gravity has the same effect on arterial and venous pressures and thus does not change the *arteriovenous pressure difference* at any one height level. There

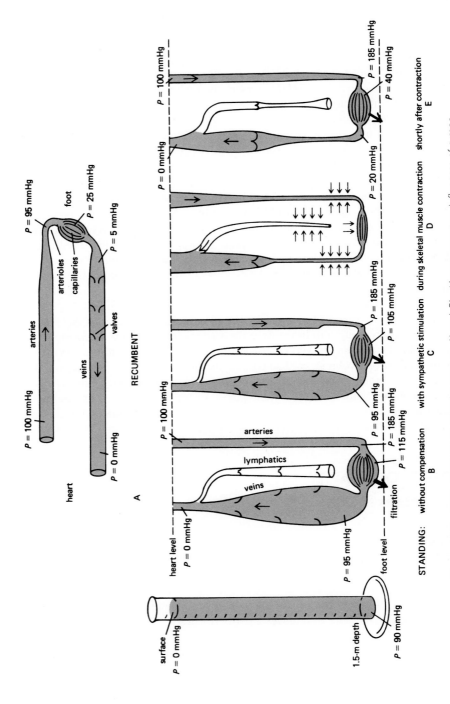

Figure 11-2 Effect of gravity on vascular pressure (A and B) with compensatory influences of sympathetic stimulation (C) and the skeletal muscle pump (D and E).

are, however, two major direct effects of the increased pressure in the lower extremities that are shown in Fig. 11-2*B*: (1) the absolute increase in venous pressure distends peripheral veins and greatly increases peripheral venous volume, and (2) the absolute increase in capillary hydrostatic pressure causes a tremendously high transcapillary filtration rate.

For reasons to be described, a reflex activation of sympathetic nerves accompanies the transition from a recumbent to an upright position. However, Fig. 11-2*C* shows how vasoconstriction from sympathetic activation is only marginally effective in ameliorating the adverse effects of gravity on the lower extremities. Arteriolar constriction can cause a greater pressure drop across arterioles, but this has only a limited effect on capillary pressure because venous pressure remains extremely high. Filtration will continue at a very high rate. In fact, the normal cardiovascular reflex mechanisms alone are incapable of dealing with upright posture without the aid of the "skeletal muscle pump." A person who remained upright without intermittent contraction of the skeletal muscles in the legs would lose consciousness in 10 to 20 min because of the decreased brain blood flow that would stem from diminished central blood volume, stroke volume, cardiac output, and arterial pressure.

The effectiveness of the skeletal muscle pump in counteracting venous blood pooling and edema formation in the lower extremities during standing is illustrated in Fig. 11-2*D* and *E*. The compression of vessels during skeletal muscle contraction expels both venous blood and lymphatic fluid from the lower extremities (Fig. 11-2*D*). Immediately after a skeletal muscle contraction, both veins and lymphatic vessels are relatively empty because their one-way valves prevent the back flow of previously expelled fluid (Fig. 11-2*E*). Most important, the weight of the venous and lymphatic fluid columns is temporarily supported by the closed one-way valve leaflets. Consequently, venous pressure is drastically lowered immediately after skeletal muscle contraction and rises only gradually as veins refill with blood from the capillaries. Thus capillary pressure and transcapillary fluid filtration rate are dramatically reduced for some period after a skeletal muscle contraction. Periodic skeletal muscle contractions can keep the average value of venous pressure at levels that are only moderately above normal. This, in combination with an increased pressure drop across vasoconstricted arterioles, prevents capillary pressures from rising to intolerable levels in the lower extremities. Some transcapillary fluid filtration is still present, but the increased lymphatic flow resulting from the skeletal muscle pump is normally sufficient to prevent severe edema formation in the feet.

The actions of the skeletal muscle pump, however beneficial, do not completely prevent a rise in the average venous pressure and blood pooling in the lower extremities on standing. Thus, assuming an upright position upsets the cardiovascular system and elicits reflex cardiovascular adjustments, as shown in Fig. 11-3.

As with all cardiovascular responses, the key to understanding the alterations associated with standing is to distinguish the primary disturbances from the compensatory responses. As shown in the top part of Fig. 11-3, the immedi-

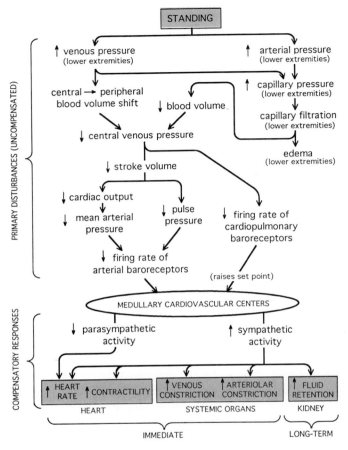

Figure 11-3 Cardiovascular mechanisms involved when changing from a recumbent to a standing position.

ate consequence of standing is an increase in both arterial and venous pressure in the lower extremities. By the chain of events shown, the primary disturbances influence the cardiovascular centers by lessening the normal input from both the arterial and the cardiopulmonary baroreceptors.

The result of a decreased baroreceptor input to the cardiovascular centers will be reflex adjustments appropriate to increase blood pressure—i.e., decreased cardiac parasympathetic nerve activity and increased activity of the cardiovascular sympathetic nerves as shown in the bottom part of Fig. 11-3. Heart rate and cardiac contractility will increase, as will arteriolar and venous constriction in most systemic organs (brain and heart excepted).

Heart rate and total peripheral resistance are higher when an individual stands than when the individual is lying down. Note that these particular cardiovascular variables are not directly influenced by standing but *are* changed by the compensatory responses. Stroke volume and cardiac output, conversely, are usually decreased below their recumbent values during quiet standing despite the reflex adjustments that tend to increase them. This is because the reflex adjustments do not quite overcome the primary disturbance on these variables caused by standing. This is in keeping with the general dictum that short-term cardiovascular compensations are never quite complete.

Mean arterial pressure is often found to increase when a person changes from the recumbent to the standing position. At first glance, this is a violation of many rules of cardiovascular system operation. How can a compensation be more than complete? Moreover, how is increased sympathetic activity compatible with higher than normal mean arterial pressure in the first place? In the case of standing, there are many answers to these apparent puzzles. First, the average arterial baroreceptor discharge rate can actually decrease in spite of a small increase in mean arterial pressure *if* there is simultaneously a sufficiently large decrease in pulse pressure. Second, mean arterial pressure determined by sphygmomanometry from the arm of a standing individual *overestimates* the mean arterial pressure actually being sensed by the baroreceptors in the carotid sinus region of the neck because of gravitational effects. Third, the influence on the medullary cardiovascular centers from cardiopulmonary receptors may raise the arterial pressure by mechanisms shown in Fig. 10-7A.

The kidney is especially susceptible to changes in sympathetic nerve activity, and consequently, as shown in Fig. 11-3, every reflex alteration in sympathetic activity has influences on fluid balance that become important in the long term. Standing, which is associated with an increase in sympathetic tone, ultimately results in an increase in fluid volume. The ultimate benefit of this is that an increase in blood volume generally reduces the magnitude of the reflex alterations required to tolerate upright posture.

Responses to Zero Gravity

The cardiovascular system of an individual who travels outside of the earth's atmosphere undergoes a variety of adaptive changes to zero gravity. The time course of the alterations as well as the underlying cellular ramifications are poorly understood, but the consequences of these changes are substantial enough that international efforts are being made to obtain more precise information.

The most significant immediate change that occurs on entering a gravity-free environment is a shift of fluid from the lower extremities to the upper portions of the body. The consequences of this shift include distention of the head and neck veins, facial edema, nasal stuffiness, and decreases in calf girth and leg volume. In addition, the increase in central blood volume stimulates the cardiopulmonary mechanoreceptors which influence renal function by neural and hormonal pathways to promote fluid loss. The individual begins to lose weight and, within a few days, becomes hypovolemic (by earth standards).

Several other cardiovascular changes during space flight have been noted for which mechanisms are not clearly understood. These include increases in resting heart rate, arterial pulse pressure, and the incidence of cardiac arrhythmias. The increase in heart rate is the opposite of that which would be expected from cardiopulmonary baroreflexes in this situation. The increase in arterial pulse pressure may reflect increased stroke volume as a result of increased cardiac filling pressure (the Frank-Starling law). The increased incidence of arrhythmias could be related to a sympathetic/parasympathetic neural imbalance and/or the significant fluid, electrolyte, and hormonal changes which are occurring. In general, however, the cardiovascular system appears to adapt quite effectively to the novel situation of zero gravity.

Upon reentry into the gravitational field, space travelers invariably suffer to some degree from *orthostatic* or *postural hypotension,* i.e., the transient fall in blood pressure that occurs in response to standing up is exaggerated. This appears to be due primarily to the decrease in circulating blood volume which occurs in space. Reversal of the zero gravity-induced alterations may take as long as three weeks to be accomplished. Efforts made in space to diminish the cardiovascular changes (including exercise programs, lower body negative pressure devices, and salt and water loading) have met with limited success.

For those of us who remain earthbound, it is pertinent to note that many of the changes that occur at zero gravity are identical to those that occur in individuals subjected to long-term bed rest. In such individuals, gravitational influences are minimized because of the recumbent position. Blood shifts from the veins in the legs to the central venous pool and body fluid-reduction mechanisms are evoked. The decrease in circulating blood volume makes these individuals susceptible to orthostatic hypotension, a common problem for patients who are just resuming an ambulatory state. (See also Study Questions 51 to 54.)

EFFECT OF EXERCISE

Responses to Acute Exercise

Physical exercise is one of the most ordinary yet taxing situations with which the cardiovascular system must cope. The specific alterations in cardiovascular function that occur during exercise depend on several factors including: (1) the type of exercise—i.e., whether it is predominantly "dynamic" (rhythmic or isotonic) or "static" (isometric); (2) the intensity and duration of the exercise; (3) the age of the individual; and (4) the level of "fitness" of the individual. The example shown in Fig. 11-4 is typical of the cardiovascular alterations that might occur in a normal, untrained, middle-aged adult doing a dynamic-type exercise such as running or dancing. Note especially that heart rate and cardiac output increase greatly during exercise and that mean arterial pressure and pulse pressure also increase significantly. These alterations ensure that the increased metabolic demands of the exercising skeletal muscle are met by appropriate increases in skeletal muscle blood flow.

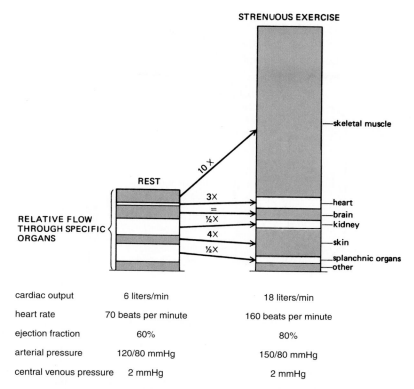

Figure 11-4   Cardiovascular adjustments to strenuous exercise.

Many of the adjustments to exercise are due to a large increase in sympathetic activity, which results from the mechanisms outlined in Fig. 11-5. One of the primary disturbances associated with the stress and/or anticipation of exercise originates within the cerebral cortex and exerts an influence on the medullary cardiovascular centers through corticohypothalamic pathways. This set-point-raising influence, referred to as the "central command," acts on the neural portion of the arterial baroreceptor system and causes mean arterial pressure to be regulated to a higher than normal level, as discussed in Chap. 10 (see Fig. 10-7A). Also indicated in Fig. 11-5 is the possibility that a second set-point-raising influence may reach the cardiovascular centers from chemoreceptors in the active skeletal muscles. Such an input would also contribute to the elevations in sympathetic activity and mean arterial pressure that accompany exercise.

A major disturbance on the cardiovascular system during dynamic exercise, however, is the great decrease in total peripheral resistance caused by metabolic vasodilator accumulation and decreased vascular resistance in active skeletal muscle. As indicated in Fig. 11-5, decreased total peripheral resistance is a pres-

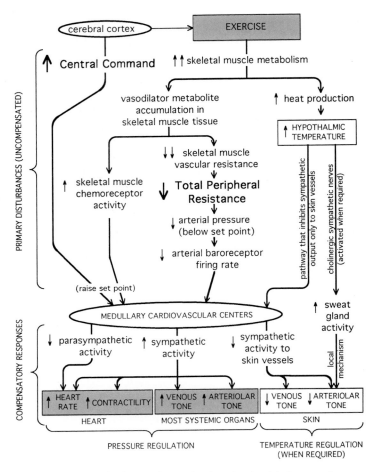

Figure 11-5   Cardiovascular mechanisms involved during exercise.

sure-lowering disturbance that elicits a strong increase in sympathetic activity through the arterial baroreceptor reflex (see Fig. 10-7B).

Although mean arterial pressure is above normal during exercise, the decreased total peripheral resistance causes it to fall below the elevated level to which it would be regulated by the set-point-raising influences on the cardiovascular center alone. As shown in Fig. 10-7B, the arterial baroreceptor reflex pathway responds to this circumstance with a large increase in sympathetic activity. Thus the arterial baroreceptor reflex is responsible for a large portion of the increase in sympathetic activity that accompanies exercise despite the seemingly contradictory fact that arterial pressure is higher than normal. In fact, were it not for the arterial baroreceptor reflex, the decrease in total peripheral resistance that occurs during exercise would cause mean arterial pressure to fall well below normal.

As discussed in Chap. 10, and indicated in Figs. 11-4 and 11-5, cutaneous blood flow may increase during exercise despite a generalized increase in sympathetic vasoconstrictor tone because thermal reflexes can override pressure reflexes in the special case of skin blood flow control. Temperature reflexes, of course, are usually activated during strenuous exercise to dissipate the excess heat being produced by the active skeletal muscles. Often cutaneous flow decreases at the onset of exercise (as part of the generalized increase in arteriolar tone from increased sympathetic vasoconstrictor activity) and then increases later during exercise as body heat and temperature build up.

In addition to the increases in skeletal muscle and skin blood flow, coronary blood flow increases substantially during strenuous exercise. This is primarily due to local metabolic vasodilation of coronary arterioles as a result of increased cardiac work and myocardial oxygen consumption.

Two important mechanisms that participate in the cardiovascular response to dynamic exercise are not shown in Fig. 11-5. The first is the skeletal muscle pump, which was discussed in connection with upright posture. The skeletal muscle pump is a very important factor in promoting venous return during exercise and thus preventing the increased heart rate and cardiac contractility from drastically lowering central venous pressure. The second factor is the respiratory pump which also promotes venous return during exercise. Exaggerated respiratory movements that occur during exercise increase the effectiveness of the respiratory pump and thus enhance venous return and cardiac filling.

As indicated in Fig. 11-4, the average central venous pressure does not change much, if at all, during strenuous dynamic exercise. This is because the cardiac output and the venous return curves are both shifted upward during exercise. Thus the cardiac output and venous return will be elevated without a significant change in central venous pressure. (Review Fig. 9-5.)

In summary, the profound cardiovascular adjustments to dynamic exercise shown in Fig. 11-5 all occur automatically as a consequence of the operation of the normal cardiovascular control mechanisms. The tremendous increase in skeletal muscle blood flow is accomplished largely by increased cardiac output but also in part by diverting flow away from the kidneys and the splanchnic organs.

Static (i.e., isometric) exercise presents a much different disturbance on the cardiovascular system than does dynamic exercise. As discussed in the previous section, dynamic exercise produces large reductions in total peripheral resistance because of local metabolic vasodilation in exercising muscles. Static efforts, even of moderate intensity, cause a compression of the vessels in the contracting muscles and a reduction in the blood flow through them. Thus, total peripheral resistance does not usually fall during static exercise and may even increase significantly if several large muscles are involved. The primary disturbances on the cardiovascular system during static exercise seem to be set-point-raising inputs to the medullary cardiovascular centers from the cerebral cortex (central command) and chemoreceptors in the contracting muscle.

Cardiovascular effects of static exercise include increases in heart rate, cardiac output, and arterial pressure, all of which are the result of increases in sympathetic drive. Static exercise, however, produces less of an increase in heart rate and cardiac output and more of an increase in diastolic, systolic, and mean arterial pressure than does dynamic exercise. Because of the higher afterload on the heart during static exercise, cardiac work is significantly higher than during dynamic exercise.

The time course of recovery of the various cardiovascular variables after a bout of exercise depends on many factors including the type, duration, and intensity of the exercise as well as the overall fitness of the individual. Muscle blood flow normally returns to a resting value within a few minutes after dynamic exercise. However, if an arterial constriction prevents a normal *active hyperemia* from occurring during dynamic exercise, the recovery will take much longer than normal. After isometric exercise, muscle blood flow often rises to near maximum levels before returning to normal with a time course which varies with the duration and intensity of the effort. Part of the increase in muscle blood flow which follows isometric exercise might be classified as *reactive hyperemia* in response to the blood flow restriction caused by compressional forces within the muscle during the exercise. (See also Study Questions 55 to 58 and 60.)

Responses to Chronic Exercise

Physical training or "conditioning" produces substantial beneficial effects on the cardiovascular system. The specific alterations that occur depend on the type of exercise, the intensity and duration of the training period, the age of the individual, and his or her original level of fitness.

In general, however, repeated physical exercise over a period of several weeks is associated with an increase in the individual's work capacity. Cardiovascular alterations associated with conditioning may include increases in circulating blood volume, decreases in heart rate, increases in cardiac stroke volume, and decreases in arterial blood pressure during both resting and exercising states. These changes produce a general decrease in myocardial oxygen demand and an increase in the *cardiac reserve* (potential for increasing cardiac output) that can be called on during times of stress. Ventricular chamber enlargement often accompanies dynamic exercise conditioning regimes (endurance training) whereas increases in myocardial mass and ventricular wall thickness are more pronounced with static exercise conditioning regimes (strength training). These structural alterations improve the pumping capabilities of the myocardium.[2] Deconditioning occurs with the cessation of the exercise program and the changes rapidly reverse.

---

[2] However, as will be described in the next chapter, ventricular chamber enlargement and myocardial hypertrophy are not always hallmarks of improved cardiac performance but may be adaptive responses to various pathological states which, if extreme, may not be helpful.

It is not clear as yet whether physical conditioning per se can actually prevent or delay the development of coronary artery disease. While the studies to date have not established cause and effect, there seems to be a positive correlation between physical activity and a decreased incidence of coronary heart disease in humans. It is increasingly evident that recovery from a myocardial infarction or cardiac surgery is enhanced by an appropriate increase in physical activity. The benefits of cardiac rehabilitation programs may be partially dependent on exercise-induced psychological alterations that produce an overall sense of well-being.

EFFECT OF AGING

Aging is a normal process. Everyone inevitably undergoes certain predictable, irreversible physiological changes that are part of a continuum beginning at birth. The changes that occur in late adulthood are often thought to be the result of the cumulative effect of "errors" that cause a generalized deterioration of the individual (the "wear and tear" theory). However, it is more likely that the aging process is under some sort of genetic control and that elimination of all disease processes will not expand our maximum life span much beyond our current limit of about 100 years.

In general, as we get older, we get slower, stiffer, and drier. Connective tissue becomes less elastic, capillary density decreases in many tissues, mitotic activity of dividing cells becomes slower, and fixed postmitotic cells (such as nerve and muscle fibers) are lost. While these changes do not, in general, alter the basic physiological processes, they do have an influence upon the rate at which various homeostatic mechanisms operate.

Age-dependent changes that occur in the heart include: (1) a decrease in the resting and maximum cardiac index, (2) a decrease in the maximum heart rate, (3) an increase in the contraction and relaxation time of the heart muscle, (4) an increase in the myocardial stiffness during diastole, and (5) an accumulation of pigment in the myocardial cells. Changes that occur in the vascular bed with age include a decrease in capillary density in some tissues, a decrease in arterial compliance, and an increase in total peripheral vascular resistance. These changes combine to produce the age-dependent increases in arterial pulse pressure and mean arterial pressure which were discussed in Chap. 7. The increases in arterial pressure impose a greater afterload upon the heart, and this may be partially responsible for the age-dependent decreases in cardiac index.

Arterial baroreceptor-induced responses to changes in blood pressure are blunted with age. This is due in part to a decrease in afferent activity from the arterial baroreceptors because of the age-dependent increase in arterial rigidity. In addition, the total amount of norepinephrine contained in the sympathetic nerve endings of the myocardium decreases with age, and the myocardial responsiveness to catecholamines declines. Thus the efferent component of the reflex is also compromised. These changes may partially account for the apparent age-dependent sluggishness in the responses to postural changes and recovery from exercise.

It is important (although often difficult) to separate age-dependent alterations from disease-induced changes in physiological function. Cardiovascular diseases are the major cause of death in an aging population. Atherosclerosis and hypertension are the primary culprits in our society. These "diseases" lack the universality necessary to be categorized as aging processes but generally occur with increasing incidence in the older population. Pharmacological interventions and reduction of risk factors (smoking, obesity, high fat or high sodium diets, inactivity) by modification of life style can alter the incidence intensity, and progression of these diseases. It is also possible that some of the previously mentioned interventions may prevent early expression of some of the normal aging processes and prolong the life span of a given individual. No practical intervention, however, is currently available that will increase the maximum potential life span of humans.

Study Questions: 51 to 60

12

CARDIOVASCULAR FUNCTION IN PATHOLOGICAL SITUATIONS

OBJECTIVES

The student understands the primary disturbances, compensatory responses, decompensatory processes, and possible therapeutic interventions that pertain to various abnormal cardiovascular situations.

1   Defines circulatory shock.
2   Identifies the primary disturbances that can account for cardiogenic, hypovolemic, anaphylactic, septic, and neurogenic shock states.
3   Lists the compensatory processes that may arise during shock and describes how these lead to irreversible shock states.
4   Identifies the decompensatory processes that may arise during shock and describes how these lead to irreversible shock states.
5   Indicates how coronary artery disease may lead to abnormal cardiac function.
6   Defines the term *angina pectoris* and describes the mechanisms that promote its development.
7   Indicates the mechanisms by which various therapeutic interventions may alleviate angina and myocardial ischemia in association with coronary artery disease.
8   Defines the term *heart failure.*
9   Identifies the short-term and long-term compensatory processes that accompany heart failure.
10   Describes the benefits and detriments of the fluid accumulation that accompanies heart failure.
11   Defines *hypertension.*
12   Identifies the various factors that may contribute to the development of primary hypertension.
13   Describes the role of the kidney in establishing and/or maintaining hypertension.

In this last chapter, we will introduce some of the pathological situations that can interfere with the homeostatic functions of the cardiovascular system. It is not intended as an in-depth coverage of cardiovascular diseases but rather as an introductory presentation of how the physiological processes described previously are evoked and/or altered during various abnormal cardiovascular states. In each case there is generally a primary disturbance that evokes appropriate compensatory reflex responses. Often, however, pathological situations also lead to inappropriate "decompensatory processes" which tend to accelerate the deterioration of cardiovascular function. Therapeutic interventions may be required and are often designed to limit or reverse these decompensatory processes.

CIRCULATORY SHOCK

A state of circulatory shock exists whenever there is a generalized, severe reduction in blood supply to the body tissues. Even with all cardiovascular compensatory mechanisms activated, arterial pressure is usually (though not always) low in shock.

Primary Disturbances

In general, the shock state is precipitated by either severely depressed myocardial functional ability or by grossly inadequate cardiac filling. The former situation is called *cardiogenic shock* and occurs whenever cardiac pumping ability is compromised (e.g., severe arrhythmias, abrupt valve misfunction, coronary occlusions, and myocardial infarction). The latter situation can be caused by any number of conditions that decrease central venous volume:

1   *Hypovolemic shock* accompanies significant hemorrhage (usually greater than 20 percent of blood volume), severe burns, chronic diarrhea, or prolonged vomiting. These situations can induce shock by depleting body fluids and thus circulating blood volume.
2   *Anaphylactic shock* occurs as a result of a severe allergic reaction to an antigen to which the patient has developed a sensitivity (e.g., insect bites, antibiotics, foodstuffs). This immunological event, also called an "immediate hypersensitivity reaction," is mediated by several substances (such as histamine, prostaglandins, leukotrienes, bradykinin) that, by multiple mechanisms not well understood, result in substantial peripheral vasodilation.
3   *Septic shock* is caused by vasodilator effects of substances released by infective agents. One of the most common is *endotoxin,* a lipopolysaccharide released from bacteria. This substance induces the formation of a nitric oxide synthase (called *inducible* NO synthase to distinguish it from the normally present *constitutive* NO synthase) in endothelial cells, vascular smooth muscle, and macrophages which then produce large amounts of the vasodilator, nitric oxide.
4   *Neurogenic shock* is produced by loss of vascular tone due to inhibition of the normal tonic activity of the sympathetic vasoconstrictor nerves and often

occurs with deep general anesthesia or in reflex response to deep pain associated with traumatic injuries. The transient vasovagal syncope that may be evoked by strong emotions is a mild form of neurogenic shock.

As shown in the top half of Fig. 12-1, the common primary disturbances in all forms of shock are decreased cardiac output and decreased mean arterial pressure. Generally, the reduction in arterial pressure is substantial, and so therefore is the influence on the cardiovascular centers from reduced arterial baroreceptor discharge rate. In addition, in the case of hypovolemic, anaphylactic, and septic shock, diminished activity of the cardiopulmonary baroreceptors due to a decrease in central venous pressure and/or volume acts on the medullary cardiovascular centers to stimulate sympathetic output.[1] If arterial pressure falls below about 60 mmHg, brain blood flow begins to fall and this elicits the cerebral ischemic response. As indicated in Chap. 10, the cerebral ischemic response causes the most intense of all activation of the sympathetic nerves.

Compensatory Mechanisms

In general, the various forms of shock elicit the compensatory responses in the autonomic nervous system that we would expect from a fall in blood pressure.[2] These are indicated in the bottom half of Fig. 12-1. These compensatory responses to shock, however, may be much more intense than those that accompany more ordinary cardiovascular disturbances. Many of the commonly recognized symptoms of shock (e.g., pallor, cold clammy skin, rapid heart rate, muscle weakness, venous constriction) are a result of these autonomic neural compensatory processes. When these immediate compensatory processes are inadequate, the individual may also show signs of abnormally low arterial pressure, such as dizziness, confusion, or loss of consciousness.

There are some additional compensatory processes that are initiated during the shock state:

1   Breathing is rapid and shallow, which promotes venous return to the heart by action of the respiratory pump.
2   The release of renin from the kidney as a result of sympathetic stimulation promotes the formation of the hormone, angiotensin II, which is a potent vasoconstrictor and participates in the increase in total peripheral resistance even in mild shock states.

---

[1]   In the case of cardiogenic shock, central venous pressure will increase; and in the case of neurogenic shock, central venous pressure cannot be predicted since both cardiac output and venous return are likely to be depressed. Thus, in these instances, it is not clear how the cardiopulmonary baroreceptors affect autonomic output.

[2]   Two primary exceptions to this statement include (1) neurogenic shock, where reflex responses may be absent or lead to further depression of blood pressure, and (2) certain instances of cardiogenic shock associated with inferoposterior myocardial infarctions, which elicit a reflex bradycardia and decrease sympathetic drive (the Bezold-Jarisch reflex).

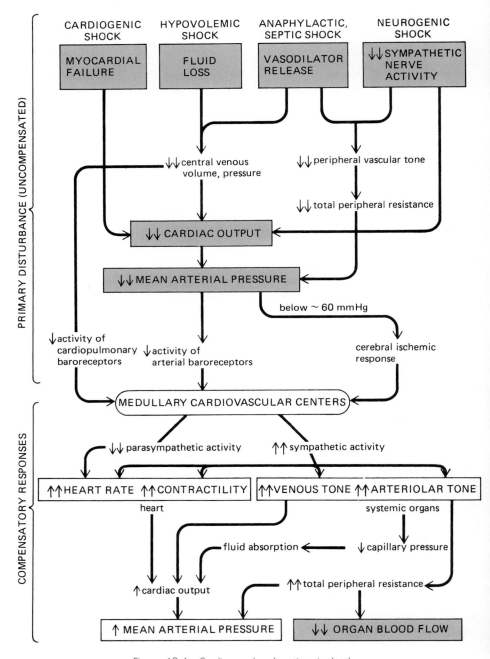

Figure 12-1   Cardiovascular alterations in shock.

3   Circulating levels of epinephrine from the adrenal medulla increase in re-
    sponse to sympathetic stimulation and contribute to the vasoconstriction.
4   The increase in arteriolar constriction reduces capillary hydrostatic pressure.
    Because plasma oncotic pressure has not changed (at least initially), there is
    a net shift of fluid from the interstitial space into the vascular space.
5   Glycogenolysis in the liver induced by epinephrine and norepinephrine re-
    sults in a release of glucose and a rise in blood (and interstitial) glucose lev-
    els and, more importantly, a rise in extracellular osmolarity by as much as 20
    mOsm. This will induce a shift of fluid from the intracellular space into the
    extracellular (including intravascular) space.

The latter two processes result in a sort of "autotransfusion" that can move as
much as 1 liter of fluid into the vascular space in the first hour after the onset of
the shock episode. This fluid shift accounts for the reduction in hematocrit that is
commonly observed in hemorrhagic shock.

   In addition to the immediate compensatory responses shown in Fig. 12-1,
fluid retention mechanisms are evoked by hypovolemic states that affect the situation in the long term. Recall that a decrease in activity of the cardiopulmonary
baroreceptors causes production and release of the antidiuretic hormone, vasopressin, from the posterior pituitary. In addition to being a potent vasoconstrictor
and contributing to the increase in total peripheral resistance in severe shock
states, this hormone promotes water retention by the kidneys. Furthermore, activation of the renin-angiotensin-aldosterone pathway promotes renal sodium retention (by aldosterone) and the thirst sensation and drinking behavior (by angiotensin II). These processes contribute to the replenishment of extracellular
fluid volume within a few days of the shock episode.

Decompensatory Processes

Often the strong compensatory responses elicited during shock are capable of
preventing drastic reductions in arterial pressure. However, because the compensatory mechanisms involve intense arteriolar vasoconstriction, perfusion of tissues other than the heart and brain may be inadequate despite nearly normal arterial pressure. For example, blood flow through organs such as the liver and
kidneys may be reduced nearly to zero by intense sympathetic activation. The
possibility of permanent renal or hepatic ischemic damage is a very real concern
even in seemingly mild shock situations. Often patients who have apparently re-
covered from a state of shock die several days later because of renal failure and
uremia.

   The immediate danger with shock is that it may enter the *progressive stage,*
wherein the general cardiovascular situation progressively degenerates, or, worse
yet, enter the *irreversible stage,* where no intervention can halt the ultimate collapse of cardiovascular function that results in death.

   The mechanisms behind progressive and irreversible shock are not completely understood. However, it is clear from the mechanisms shown in Fig.
12-2 how bodily homeostasis can progressively deteriorate with prolonged

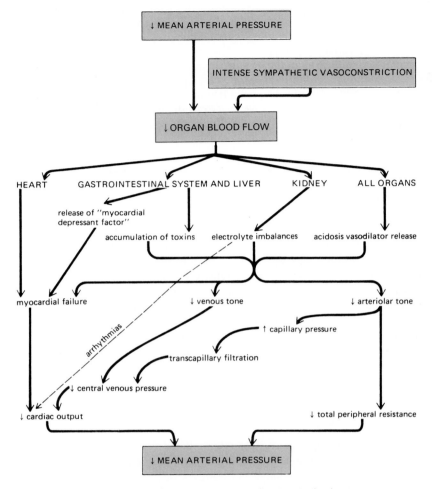

Figure 12-2   Decompensatory mechanisms in shock.

reductions in organ blood flow. These homeostatic disturbances in turn adversely affect various components of the cardiovascular system so that arterial pressure and thus organ blood flow is further reduced. Note that the events shown in Fig. 12-2 are *decompensatory mechanisms*. Reduced arterial pressure leads to alterations that further reduce arterial pressure rather than correct it. These decompensatory mechanisms that are occurring at the tissue level to lower blood pressure are eventually further compounded by a reduction in sympathetic drive and a change from vasoconstriction to vasodilation with a further lowering of blood pressure. The factors that lead to this unexpected reduction in sympathetic drive from the medullary cardiovascular centers are not clearly understood but may include activation of opiate receptors in the brain and/or afferent vagal input from various thoracic and splanchnic receptors. If the shock state is severe enough and/or has persisted long enough to enter the progressive stage, the self-reinforcing decompensatory mechanisms progressively drive arterial pressure down. Unless corrective measures are taken quickly, death will ultimately result. (See also Study Questions 61 to 63.)

CARDIAC DISTURBANCES

Coronary Artery Disease

Whenever coronary blood flow falls below that required to meet the metabolic needs of the heart, the myocardium is said to be *ischemic* and the pumping capability of the heart is impaired. The most common cause of myocardial ischemia is atherosclerotic disease of the large coronary arteries. In atherosclerotic disease, localized lipid deposits called *plaques* develop within the arterial walls. With severe disease these plaques may become so large that they physically narrow the lumen of arteries (producing a stenosis) and thus greatly and permanently increase the normally low vascular resistance of these large arteries. This extra resistance adds to the resistance of other coronary vascular segments and tends to reduce coronary flow. If the coronary artery stenosis is not too severe, local metabolic vasodilator mechanisms may reduce arteriolar resistance sufficiently to compensate for the abnormally large arterial resistance. Thus an individual with coronary artery disease may have perfectly normal coronary blood flow when resting. A coronary artery stenosis of any significance will, however, limit the extent to which coronary flow can increase above its resting value by reducing maximum achievable coronary flow. This occurs because, even with very low arteriolar resistance, the overall vascular resistance of the coronary vascular bed is high if arterial resistance is high.

Coronary artery disease can jeopardize cardiac function in several ways. Ischemic muscle cells are electrically irritable and unstable and the danger of fibrillation is enhanced. During ischemia, the normal cardiac electrical excitation pathways may be altered and often ectopic pacemaker foci develop. Electrocardiographic manifestations of myocardial ischemia can be observed in individuals with coronary artery disease during exercise stress tests. In addition, there is some evidence that platelet aggregation and clotting function may be abnormal in atherosclerotic coronary arteries and the danger of thrombus or emboli formation is enhanced. It appears that certain platelet suppressants or anticoagulants such as aspirin may be beneficial in the treatment of this consequence of coronary artery disease. (Details of the blood clotting process are included in Appendix D.)

Myocardial ischemia not only impairs the pumping ability of the heart, but also produces intense, debilitating chest pain called *angina pectoris.* Anginal pain is often absent in individuals with coronary artery disease when they are resting but is induced during physical exertion or emotional excitement. Both of these situations elicit an increase in sympathetic tone that increases myocardial oxygen consumption. Myocardial ischemia and chest pain will result if coronary blood flow cannot keep pace with the increase in myocardial metabolism.

Primary treatment of coronary artery disease (and atherosclerosis, in general) should include attempts to lower blood lipids by dietary and pharmacological techniques which prevent (and possibly reverse) further development of the plaques. The interested student should consult medical biochemistry and pharmacology texts for a complete discussion of this very important topic.

Treatment of the angina that is a *result* of coronary artery disease may involve several different pharmacological approaches. First, vasodilator drugs such as nitroglycerin may be used to acutely increase coronary blood flow. In addition to increasing myocardial oxygen delivery by dilating coronary vessels, nitrates may also reduce myocardial oxygen demand by dilating systemic veins and reducing the cardiac period and by decreasing arterial resistance and reducing the cardiac afterload. Second, beta-adrenergic blocking agents such as propranalol may be used to block the effects of cardiac sympathetic nerves on heart rate and contractility. These agents limit myocardial oxygen consumption and prevent it from increasing above the level that the compromised coronary blood flow can sustain. Third, calcium-channel-blocking agents such as verapamil may be used to dilate coronary vessels. These drugs, which block entry of calcium into the vascular smooth muscle cell, interfere with normal excitation-contraction coupling. They have been found to be most useful for treating the angina caused by vasoconstrictive spasms of large coronary arteries (Prinzmetal's angina).

Surgical interventions are now commonly used to eliminate coronary artery stenosis. In some cases, x-ray techniques can be used to visualize a radiopaque, balloon-tipped catheter as it is threaded into the coronary artery to the occluded region. Rapid inflation of the balloon squeezes the plaque against the vessel wall and improves the patency of the vessel. This technique, called coronary angioplasty, may also be effective in opening occlusions produced by intravascular clots associated with acute myocardial infarction.[3] A small tube-like device called a *stent* is sometimes implanted inside the vessel at the angioplasty site. This rigid implant is thought to promote continued patency of the vessel over a longer period than angioplasty alone. If angioplasty is inappropriate or unsuccessful, coronary bypass surgery may be performed. The stenotic coronary artery segments are bypassed by implanting parallel low-resistance pathways formed either from natural (e.g., saphenous vein or mammary artery) or artificial vessels.

Chronic Congestive Heart Failure

Heart (or cardiac, or myocardial) *failure* is said to exist whenever ventricular function is depressed through myocardial damage, insufficient coronary flow, or

---

[3]   Another method for treatment of acute myocardial infarction has been the intravascular injection of substances that dissolve blood clots such as streptokinase or tissue plasminogen activating factor.

any other condition that directly impairs the mechanical performance of heart muscle. By definition, heart failure implies a *lower than normal cardiac function curve,* that is, a reduced cardiac output at any given filling pressure. We have already discussed acute heart failure in the context of cardiogenic shock and as part of the decompensatory mechanisms operating in progressive and irreversible shock. Often, however, sustained cardiac "challenges" may induce a chronic state of heart failure. Such challenges might include (1) progressive coronary artery disease, (2) sustained elevation in cardiac afterload as that which accompanies arterial hypertension or aortic valve stenosis, or (3) reduced functional muscle mass following myocardial infarction. In some instances, external causes of cardiac failure cannot be identified and some primary myocyte abnormality is to blame. This situation is referred to as *primary cardiomyopathy.* Regardless of the precipitating cause, most forms of failure are associated eventually with a reduced myocyte function. Studies suggest that calcium sequestration by the sarcoplasmic reticulum is often reduced (leading to low intracellular calcium levels during excitation-contraction coupling) and/or affinity of troponin for calcium is often diminished (leading to reduction in myofilament crossbridge formation and contractile ability).

The primary disturbance in heart failure (acute or chronic) is depressed cardiac output and thus lowered arterial pressure. Consequently, all the compensatory responses important in shock (Fig. 12-1) are also important in heart failure. In chronic heart failure, however, the cardiovascular disturbances may not be sufficient to produce a state of shock. Moreover, long-term compensatory mechanisms are especially important in chronic heart failure.

The circumstances of chronic heart failure are well illustrated by cardiac output and venous return curves such as those shown in Fig. 12-3. The normal cardiac output and normal venous return curves intersect at point A in Fig. 12-3. A cardiac output of 5 liters/min at a central venous pressure of less than 2 mmHg is indicated by the normal operating point (A). With heart failure, the heart operates on a much lower than normal cardiac output curve. Thus heart failure alone (uncompensated) shifts the cardiovascular operation from the normal point (A) to a new position, as illustrated by point B in Fig. 12-3—i.e., cardiac output falls below normal while central venous pressure rises above normal. The decreased cardiac output leads to decreased arterial pressure and reflex activation of the cardiovascular sympathetic nerves. Increased sympathetic nerve activity tends to (1) raise the cardiac output curve toward normal and (2) increase peripheral venous pressure through venous constriction and thus raise the venous return curve above normal. Cardiovascular operation will shift from point B to point C in Fig. 12-3. Thus the depressed cardiac output is substantially improved by the immediate consequences of increased sympathetic nerve activity. Note, however, that the cardiac output at point C is still below normal. The arterial pressure associated with cardiovascular operation at point C is likely to be near normal, however, since higher than normal total peripheral resistance will accompany higher than normal sympathetic nerve activity.

In the long term, cardiovascular operation cannot remain at point C in Fig.

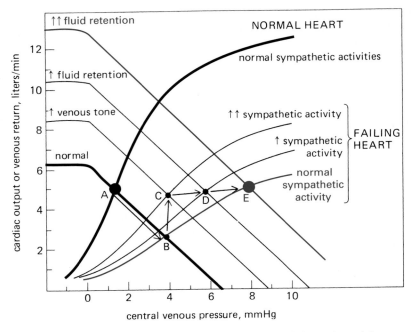

Figure 12-3   Cardiovascular alterations with compensated chronic heart failure.

12-3. Operation at point C involves higher than normal sympathetic activity, and this will inevitably cause a gradual increase in blood volume by the mechanisms that were described in Chap. 7. Over several days, there is a progressive rise in the venous return curve as a result of increased blood volume. Recall that this process involves a sympathetically induced release of renin from the kidney, which activates the renin-angiotensin-aldosterone system that promotes fluid retention. This will shift the cardiovascular operating point from C to D to E as shown in Fig. 12-3.

Note that increased fluid retention (C→D→E in Fig. 12-3) causes a progressive increase in cardiac output toward normal and simultaneously allows a *reduction in sympathetic nerve activity toward the normal value.* Reduced sympathetic activity is beneficial for several reasons. First, decreased arteriolar constriction permits renal and splanchnic blood flow to return toward more normal values. Second, myocardial oxygen consumption may fall as sympathetic nerve activity falls, even though cardiac output tends to increase. Recall that increased heart rate and increased cardiac contractility greatly increase myocardial oxygen consumption. Reduced myocardial oxygen consumption is especially beneficial in situations where inadequate coronary blood flow is the cause of the heart failure. In any case, once a normal cardiac output has been achieved, the individual is said to be in a "compensated" state.[4]

Unfortunately, the consequences of fluid retention in cardiac failure are not all beneficial. Note in Fig. 12-3 that fluid retention $(C \rightarrow D \rightarrow E)$ will cause both peripheral and central venous pressures to be much higher than their normal values. Chronically high central venous pressure causes chronically increased end-diastolic volume (cardiac dilation). Up to a point, cardiac performance is improved by increased cardiac filling volume through the Frank-Starling law. Excessive cardiac dilation, however, can impair cardiac function because increased total wall tension is required to generate pressure within an enlarged ventricular chamber $(T = P \cdot r,$ Chap. 4).

The high venous pressure associated with fluid retention also adversely affects organ function because transcapillary fluid filtration, edema formation, and congestion are produced by a high venous pressure (hence the term *congestive heart failure*). Pulmonary edema with dyspnea (shortness of breath)[5] and respiratory crisis often accompany left heart failure. Common signs of right heart failure include distended neck veins, ankle edema, and fluid accumulation in the abdomen (ascites) with liver congestion and dysfunction.[6]

In the example shown in Fig. 12-3, the depression in the cardiac output curve because of heart failure is only moderately severe. Thus, it is possible, through moderate fluid retention, to achieve a normal cardiac output with essentially normal sympathetic activity (point E). The situation at point E is relatively stable because the stimuli for further fluid retention have been removed. If, however, the heart failure is more severe, the cardiac output curve may be so depressed that normal cardiac output cannot be achieved by any amount of fluid retention. In these cases fluid retention is extremely marked, as is the elevation in venous pressure, and the adverse complications of congestion are very serious problems.

Another way of looking at the effects of cardiac failure is given in Fig. 12-4. The left ventricular pressure volume loops describing the events of a cardiac cycle from a failing heart are displaced far to the right of those from normal hearts. The untreated patient described in this figure is in serious trouble with a reduced stroke volume and ejection fraction and high filling pressure. Furthermore the

---

[4] The extracellular fluid volume remains expanded after reaching the compensated state even though sympathetic activity may have returned to near normal levels. Net fluid loss requires a period of less than normal sympathetic activity which does not occur. For reasons not well understood, the cardiopulmonary baroreceptor reflexes apparently become less responsive to the increased central venous pressure and volume associated with heart failure.

[5] Patients often complain of difficulty breathing especially during the night (paroxysmal nocturnal dyspnea). Being recumbent promotes a fluid shift from the extremities into the central venous pool and lungs making the patient's pulmonary problems worse. Such patients often sleep more comfortably when propped up.

[6] Plasma volume expansion combines with abnormal liver function to reduce the concentration of plasma proteins by as much as 30 percent. This reduction in plasma oncotic pressure contributes to the development of interstitial edema of congestive heart failure.

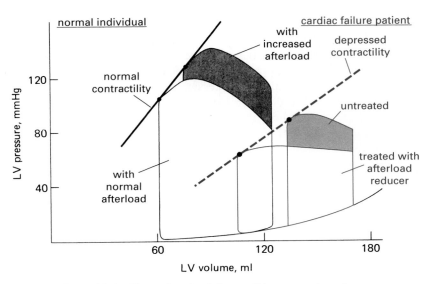

Figure 12-4   Effects of cardiac failure on LV pressure-volume loops.

slope of the line describing the end-systolic pressure volume relationship is shifted downward and is less steep indicating the reduced contractility of the cardiac muscle. However, because of this flatter relationship, small reductions in cardiac afterload will produce substantial increases in stroke volume and significantly help this patient.

As might be expected from the previous discussion, the most common symptoms of patients with congestive heart failure are associated with the inability to increase cardiac output (low exercise tolerance and fatigue) and with the compensatory fluid accumulation (shortness of breath, peripheral swelling). In severe cases, the ability of the cardiac cells to respond to increases in sympathetic stimulation is diminished by a reduction in the effective number (down-regulation) of the myocyte β_1-adrenergic receptors. This further reduces the ability of the myocytes to increase their contractility as well as the ability of the heart to increase its beating rate in response to sympathetic stimulation. Thus low maximal heart rates contribute to the reduced exercise tolerance.

Treatment of the patient with congestive failure is a difficult challenge. Treatment of the precipitating condition is of course the ideal approach, but often this cannot be done effectively. The cardiac glycosides (e.g., digitalis)[7] have been used to improve cardiac contractility (i.e., to shift the cardiac output curve upward, increasing contractile force of the myocyte at any given starting

---

[7]   A "tea" made from the leaves of the foxglove plant (digitalis purpurea) was used for centuries as a common folk remedy for the treatment of "dropsy" (congestive heart failure with significant peripheral edema). With the formal recognition of its medicinal benefits in the late eighteenth century by the English physician, Sir William Withering, digitalis became a valuable official pharmacological tool.

length).[8] These drugs are unfortunately quite toxic and often lead to unpleasant consequences.

Treatment of the congestive symptoms involves balancing the need for enhanced cardiac filling with the problems of too much fluid. Drugs that promote fluid loss (diuretics), such as furosemide or thiazides, are extremely helpful as are the angiotensin-converting enzyme (ACE) inhibitors.[9] A potent diuretic can quickly save a patient from drowning in the pulmonary exudate and reduce diastolic volume of the dilated heart to acceptable levels, but it can also lower blood pressure to dangerous levels. (See also Study Questions 64 and 65.)

HYPERTENSION

Hypertension is defined as a chronic elevation of arterial blood pressure above 140/90 mmHg for adults from 18 to 59 years of age and above 160/95 mmHg for those older than 60 years of age. It is an extremely common cardiovascular problem affecting approximately 20 percent of the adult population of the western world. It has been established beyond doubt that hypertension increases the risk of coronary artery disease, myocardial infarction, heart failure, stroke, and many other serious cardiovascular problems. Moreover, it has been clearly demonstrated that the risk of serious cardiovascular incidents is reduced by proper treatment of hypertension.

In approximately 90 percent of cases the primary abnormality that produces high blood pressure is unknown. The term *essential hypertension* is applied to this situation. In the remaining 10 percent of hypertensive patients, the cause can be traced to a variety of sources including epinephrine-producing tumors (pheochromocytomas), aldosterone-producing tumors (in primary hyperaldosteronism), certain forms of renal disease (e.g., renal artery stenosis, glomerular nephritis, toxemia of pregnancy), certain neurological disorders (e.g., brain tumors which increase intracranial pressure), certain thyroid and parathyroid disorders, aortic coarctation, lead poisoning, drug side effects, abuse of certain drugs, or even unusual dietary habits. The high blood pressure that accompanies such known causes is referred to as *secondary hypertension*. Most often, however, the true cause of the hypertension remains a mystery and it is only the symptom of high blood pressure that is treated.

---

[8] The mechanism of cardiac glycoside action is thought to involve the inhibition of the sodium/potassium adenosine triphosphatase (Na^+/K^+ ATPase) leading to increases in intracellular $[Na^+]$, which is then exchanged for extracellular calcium via the Na^+/Ca^{2+} exchanger. This results in "loading" of the sarcoplasmic reticulum during diastole and increased calcium release for subsequent excitation-contraction coupling.

[9] The ACE inhibitors are very helpful to the congestive heart failure patient for several reasons. By inhibiting the conversion of angiotensin I into its more active form, angiotensin II, peripheral vasoconstriction is reduced (which improves cardiac pumping by afterload reduction) and aldosterone levels are reduced (which promotes diuresis). In addition, ACE inhibitors also seem to prevent some of the apparently inappropriate myocyte and collagen growth that occurs with cardiac overload and failure.

In the midst of a bewildering amount of information about essential hypertension, a few universally accepted facts stand out:

1   Genetic factors contribute importantly to the development of hypertension. Familial tendencies for high blood pressure are well documented. In addition, hypertension is generally more common in males than in females, in blacks than in whites, in Chinese than in Japanese.

2   Environmental factors can influence the development of hypertension. High salt diets and/or certain forms of psychological stress may either aggravate or precipitate hypertension in genetically susceptible individuals.

3   Structural changes in the left heart and arterial vessels occur in response to hypertension. Early alterations include hypertrophy of muscle cells and thickening of the walls of the ventricle and resistance vessels. Late changes associated with deterioration of function include increases in connective tissue and loss of elasticity.

4   The established phase of hypertension is associated with an increase in total peripheral resistance. Cardiac output and/or blood volume may be elevated during the early developmental phase, but these variables are usually normal after the hypertension is established.

5   The increased total peripheral resistance associated with established hypertension may be due to (a) *rarefaction* (decrease in density) of microvessels, (b) the pronounced structural adaptations that occur in the peripheral vascular bed, (c) a continuously increased activity of the vascular smooth muscle cells[10] and/or (d) an increased sensitivity and reactivity of the vascular smooth muscle cells to external stimuli.

6   The chronic elevation in blood pressure does not appear to be due to a sustained elevation in sympathetic vasoconstrictor neural discharge nor is it due to a sustained elevation of any blood-borne vasoconstrictive factor. (Both neural and hormonal influences, however, may help to initiate primary hypertension.)

7   Blood pressure-regulating reflexes (both the short-term arterial and cardiopulmonary baroreceptor reflexes and the long-term, renal-dependent, pressure-regulating reflexes) become adapted or "reset" to regulate blood pressure at a higher than normal level.

8   Disturbances in renal function contribute importantly to the development and maintenance of primary hypertension. Recall that the urine output rate is influenced by arterial pressure, and, in the long term, arterial pressure can stabilize only at the level that makes urine output rate equal to fluid intake rate. As shown by point N in Fig. 12-5, this pressure is approximately 100 mmHg in a normal individual.

All forms of hypertension involve an alteration somewhere in the chain of events through which changes in arterial pressure produce changes in urine output rate (see Fig. 10-8) such that the renal function curve is shifted rightward as

---

10   Continuous activation of vascular smooth muscle might be evoked by autoregulatory responses to increased blood pressure, as discussed in Chap. 7. A *total body autoregulation* could produce an increase in total peripheral resistance so that total systemic flow (i.e., cardiac output) would remain nearly normal in the presence of increased mean arterial pressure.

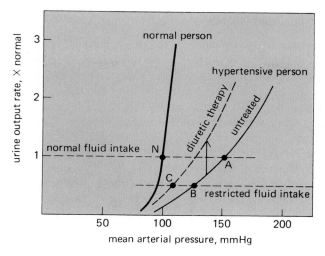

Figure 12-5   Renal function curves in hypertension and hypertension therapy.

indicated in Fig. 12-5. The important feature to note is that *higher than normal arterial pressure is required to produce a normal urine output rate in hypertension.* While this condition is always present with hypertension, it is not clear whether it could be the common cause of hypertension or simply another one of the many adaptations to it.

Consider that the untreated hypertensive individual in Fig. 12-5 would have a very low urine output rate at the normal mean arterial pressure of 100 mmHg. Recall from Fig. 10-7 that whenever the fluid intake rate exceeds the urine output rate, fluid volume must rise and consequently so will cardiac output and mean arterial pressure. With a normal fluid intake rate, this untreated hypertensive patient will ultimately stabilize at point A (mean arterial pressure = 150 mmHg). Recall from Chap. 10 that the baroreceptors adapt within days so that they have a normal discharge rate at the *prevailing* average arterial pressure. Thus, once the hypertensive individual has been at point A for a week or more, even the baroreceptor mechanism will begin resisting acute changes from the 150-mmHg pressure level.

A most important fact to realize is that, although high blood pressure must always ultimately be sustained by either high cardiac output or high total peripheral resistance, neither need be the primary cause. A shift in the relationship between arterial pressure and urine output rate, as illustrated in Fig. 12-5, however, will always produce hypertension. The possibility that the kidneys actually "set" the blood pressure is supported by evidence accumulating from kidney transplant studies. In these studies, the blood pressure is shown to "follow" the kidney (i.e., putting a hypertensive kidney in a normotensive individual produces a hypertensive individual whereas putting a normotensive kidney in a hypertensive individual produces a normotensive individual).

Therapeutic Interventions

In certain hypertensive individuals, restricting salt intake produces a substantial reduction in blood pressure because of the reduced requirement for water retention to osmotically balance the salt load. In the example of Fig. 12-5, this effect is illustrated by a shift from point A to point B. The efficacy of lowering salt intake to lower arterial pressure depends heavily on the slope of the renal function curve in the hypertensive individual. The arterial pressure of a normal individual, for example, is affected only slightly by changes in salt intake because the normal renal function curve is so steep.

A second common treatment of hypertension is diuretic therapy. Many diuretic drugs are available, but most have the effect of inhibiting renal tubular salt (and therefore fluid) reabsorption. The net effect of diuretic therapy, as shown in Fig. 12-5, is that the urine output rate for a given arterial pressure is increased; i.e., diuretic therapy raises the renal function curve. The combined result of restricted fluid intake and diuretic therapy for the hypertensive individual of Fig. 12-5 is illustrated by point C.

Other therapeutic interventions may include treatment with *α-adrenergic receptor blocking agents,* which prevent the vasoconstrictive effects of catecholamines, or *β-adrenergic blocking agents* (such as propranolol) that inhibit sympathetic influences on the heart and renal renin release. The latter approach is most successful in hypertensive patients who have high circulating renin levels. The *ACE inhibitors,* which prevent the formation of the vasoconstrictor, angiotensin II, may also be helpful under these conditions. *Calcium channel blockers,* which directly act to decrease vascular smooth muscle tone, may also be used to treat hypertension. *Alterations in life style,* including reduction of stress, decreases in caloric intake, limitation of the amount of saturated fats in the diet, and establishment of a regular exercise program, may help to reduce blood pressure in certain individuals. (See also Study Questions 61 and 62.)

Study Questions: 61 to 66

STUDY QUESTIONS

Q-1 Whenever skeletal muscle blood flow increases, blood flow to other organs must decrease. True or false?

Q-2 **a** Determine the vascular resistance of a resting skeletal muscle from the following data:

Mean arterial pressure = 100 mm Hg
Mean venous pressure = 0 mmHg
Blood flow to the muscle = 5 ml/min

b Assume that when the muscle is exercising, the resistance vessels dilate so that their internal radius doubles. If blood pressure does not change, what is the blood flow through the exercising muscle?
c What is the vascular resistance of this exercising skeletal muscle?

Q-3 Calculate the cardiac output from the following data:

Pulmonary arterial pressure = 20 mmHg
Pulmonary venous pressure = 0 mm Hg
Pulmonary vascular resistance = 4 mmHg · min/liter

Q-4 Determine the rate of glucose uptake by an exercising skeletal muscle $(\dot{G}_m)$ from the following data:

Arterial blood glucose concentration, $[G]_a = 50$ mg per 100 ml

Muscle venous blood glucose concentration, $[G]_v = 30$ mg per 100 ml

Blood flow, $\dot{Q} = 60$ ml/min

Q-5 Determine the direction of transcapillary fluid movement $(\dot{F})$ within a tissue, given the following data:

Capillary hydrostatic pressure, $P_c = 28$ mmHg
Plasma oncotic pressure, $\pi_c = 24$ mmHg
Tissue hydrostatic pressure, $P_i = -4$ mmHg
Tissue oncotic pressure, $\pi_i = 0$ mmHg

Q-6   Which of the following conditions favor edema formation?
    a Lymphatic blockage
    b Thrombophlebitis (venous clot)
    c Decreased plasma protein concentration
    d Greatly increased capillary pore size

Q-7   **a** What will happen to the potassium equilibrium potential of cardiac muscle cells when interstitial $[K^+]$ (i.e., $[K^+]_o$) is elevated?
    b What effect will this have on the cells' resting membrane potential?
    c What effect will this have on the cells' excitability?

Q-8   Very high sympathetic neural activity to the heart can lead to tetanic contraction of the cardiac muscle. True or false?

Q-9   A drug that blocks calcium channels in cardiac muscle cell membranes would be expected to decrease myocardial contractility. True or false?

Q-10   An increase in which of the following (with the others held constant) will result in an increase in the amount of active shortening of a cardiac muscle cell
    a preload
    b afterload
    c contractility

Q-11   If pulmonary artery pressure is 24/8 mmHg (systolic/diastolic), what are the respective systolic and diastolic pressures of the right ventricle?

Q-12   Because pulmonary artery pressure is so much lower than aortic pressure, the right ventricle has a larger stroke volume than the left ventricle. True or false?

Q-13   Which of the following interventions will increase cardiac stroke volume?
    a Increased ventricular filling pressure
    b Decreased arterial pressure
    c Increased activity of cardiac sympathetic nerves
    d Increased circulating catecholamine levels

Q-14   Given the following information, calculate cardiac output:
    Systemic arterial blood O_2 concentration, $[O_2]_{SA} = 200$ ml/liter
    Pulmonary arterial blood O_2 concentration, $[O_2]_{PA} = 140$ ml/liter
    Total body O_2 consumption, $\dot{V}_{O_2} = 600$ ml/min

Q-15   In which direction will cardiac output change if central venous pressure is lowered while cardiac sympathetic tone is increased?

Q-16   Increases in sympathetic neural activity to the heart will result in an increase in stroke volume by causing a decrease in end-systolic volume for any given end-diastolic volume. True or false?

Q-17 A decrease in atrioventricular nodal conduction velocity will
    a   Decrease heart rate
    b   Increase P wave amplitude
    c   Increase the PR interval
    d   Widen the QRS complex
    e   Increase ST segment duration

Q-18 If the R wave is upright and equally large on leads II and III, what is the mean electrical axis of the heart?

Q-19 Which of the following arrhythmias might result in a reduced stroke volume?
    a   Paroxysmal atrial tachycardia
    b   Ventricular tachycardia
    c   Atrial fibrillation
    d   Ventricular fibrillation
    e   Third-degree heart block

Q-20 Describe the primary pressure abnormalities associated with
    a   Aortic stenosis
    b   Mitral stenosis

Q-21 You notice an abnormally large pulsation of your patient's jugular vein which occurs at about the same time as heart sound S_1. What is your diagnosis?

Q-22 What alteration in jugular venous pulsations might accompany third-degree heart block?

Q-23 If the left ventricular chamber is enlarged, the wall tension required to generate a given systolic pressure is increased. True or false?

Q-24 Assume that three vessels with identical dimensions are combined into a network of one vessel followed by a parallel combination of the other two and that a pressure (P_i) is applied to the inlet of the first vessel while a lower pressure (P_o) exists at the outlet of the parallel pair.
    a   Find the overall resistance of the network (R_n) if the resistance of each vessel is equal to R_e.
    b   Is the pressure (P_j) at the central junction of the network closer to P_i or P_o?
    c   Use the basic flow equation to derive an equation which relates the pressure drop across the input vessel $(P_i - P_j)$ to the total pressure drop across the network $(P_i - P_o)$.

Q-25   Given the following data, calculate an individual's total peripheral resistance:

Mean arterial pressure, $\bar{P}_A = 100$ mmHg
Central venous pressure, $P_{CV} = 0$ mmHg
Cardiac output, CO = 6 liters/min

Q-26   The total peripheral resistance to blood flow is greater than the resistance to flow through any of the systemic organs. True or false?

Q-27   Other factors being equal, a decrease in the renal vascular resistance will increase TPR. True or false?

Q-28   Constriction of arterioles in an organ promotes reabsorption of interstitial fluid from that organ. True or false?

Q-29   Chronic elevation of arterial pressure requires that either cardiac output or total peripheral resistance (or both) be chronically elevated. True or false?

Q-30   Whenever cardiac output is increased, mean arterial pressure *must* also be increased. True or false?

Q-31   Acute increases in arterial pulse pressure usually result from increases in stroke volume. True or false?

Q-32   An increase in total peripheral resistance increases diastolic pressure (P_D) more than systolic pressure (P_S). True or false?

Q-33   Estimate the mean arterial pressure when the measured arterial pressure is 110/70 mmHg.

Q-34   At rest your patient has a pulse rate of 70 beats per minute and an arterial blood pressure of 119/80 mmHg. During exercise on a treadmill, pulse rate is 140 beats per minute and blood pressure is 135/90 mmHg. Use this information to estimate the exercise-related changes in the following variables:
a   Stroke volume (SV)
b   Cardiac output (CO)
c   Total peripheral resistance (TPR)

Q-35   Which of the following would increase blood flow through a skeletal muscle?
a   An increase in tissue P_{CO_2}
b   An increase in tissue adenosine
c   The presence of alpha-receptor blocking drugs
d   Sympathetic activation

Q-36   Autoregulation of blood flow implies that arterial pressure is adjusted by local mechanisms to ensure constant flow through an organ. True or false?

Q-37 Coronary blood flow will normally increase when
    a Arterial pressure increases
    b Heart rate increases
    c Sympathetic activity increases
    d The heart is dilated

Q-38 The arterioles of skeletal muscle would have little or no tone in the absence of normal sympathetic vasoconstrictor fiber activity. True or false?

Q-39 A person who hyperventilates (breathes rapidly and deeply) gets dizzy. Why?

Q-40 A patient complains of severe leg pains after walking a short distance. The pains disappear after the patient rests (this symptom is called *intermittent claudication*). What might be the problem?

Q-41 How would a stenotic aortic valve influence coronary blood flow?

Q-42 What determines central venous pressure?

Q-43 According to the Frank-Starling law, cardiac output always decreases when central venous pressure decreases. True or false?

Q-44 In a steady state, venous return will be greater than cardiac output when
    a Peripheral venous pressure is higher than normal
    b Blood volume is higher than normal
    c Cardiac sympathetic nerve activity is lower than normal

Q-45 Consider the various components of the arterial baroreceptor reflex and predict whether the following variables will increase or decrease in response to a *rise* in arterial pressure.
    a Arterial baroreceptor firing rate
    b Parasympathetic activity to the heart
    c Sympathetic activity to the heart
    d Arteriolar tone
    e Venous tone
    f Peripheral venous pressure
    g Total peripheral resistance
    h Cardiac output

Q-46 Massage of the neck over the carotid sinus area in a person experiencing a bout of paroxysmal atrial tachycardia is often effective in terminating the episode. Why?

Q-47 Indicate whether mean arterial pressure, after all adjustments, is *increased* or *decreased* by the following stimuli:
 a Low O_2 in arterial blood
 b Increased intracranial pressure
 c Increased cardiac filling pressure
 d Sense of danger
 e Visceral pain

Q-48 Describe the immediate cardiovascular consequences of giving a normal person a drug that blocks α-adrenergic receptors.

Q-49 What net short-term alterations in mean arterial pressure and sympathetic activity would the following produce?
 a Blood loss through hemorrhage
 b Cutaneous pain
 c Systemic hypoxia
 d Local metabolic vasodilation in skeletal muscle

Q-50 Your patient has lower-than-normal mean arterial pressure and higher-than-normal pulse rate. Which of the following are possible diagnoses?
 a low blood volume
 b anxiety
 c a cardiac valve problem
 d elevated intracranial pressure

Q-51 How are the thin-walled capillaries able to withstand pressures greater than 100 mmHg without rupturing?

Q-52 Soldiers faint when standing at attention on a very hot day more often than on a cooler day. Why?

Q-53 For several days after an extended period of bed rest, patients often become dizzy when they stand upright quickly because of an exaggerated transient fall in arterial pressure (*orthostatic hypotension*). Why might this be so?

Q-54 Vertical immersion to the neck in tepid water produces a diuresis in many individuals. What mechanisms might account for this phenomenon?

Q-55 How is the decrease in skeletal muscle vascular resistance evident from Fig. 11-4?

Q-56 Is a decrease in total peripheral resistance implied in Fig. 11-4?

Q-57 What in Fig. 11-4 implies increased sympathetic activity?

Q-58 From the information given in Fig. 11-4,
    a Calculate the resting and exercising stroke volumes (*SV*s).
    b Calculate the resting and exercising end-diastolic volumes (*EDV*s).
    c Calculate the resting and exercising end-systolic volumes (*ESV*s).
    d Construct a sketch that indicates, as accurately as possible, how this exercise affects the left ventricular volume-pressure cycle.

Q-59 Most artificial respirators force air into the lungs with positive pressure. Respiration with such a device is detrimental to cardiovascular function. Why?

Q-60 Blood pressure can rise to extremely high levels during strenuous isometric exercise maneuvers like weight lifting. Why?

Q-61 Clinical signs of hypovolemic shock often include pale and cold skin, dry mucous membranes, weak but rapid pulse, and muscle weakness and mental disorientation or unconsciousness. What are the physiological conditions that account for these signs?

Q-62 Which of the following would be helpful to hemorrhagic shock victims?
    a Keep them on their feet
    b Warm them up
    c Give them fluids to drink
    d Maintain their blood pressure with catecholamine-type drugs

Q-63 What happens to hematocrit
    a In hypovolemic shock resulting from prolonged diarrhea?
    b In acute cardiogenic shock?
    c In septic shock?
    d With chronic bleeding?

Q-64 Why are diuretic drugs (see hypertension section) often helpful in treating patients in congestive heart failure?

Q-65 What is the potential danger of vigorous diuretic therapy for the patient in heart failure?

Q-66 Why would renal artery stenosis produce hypertension?

ANSWERS

A-1   False. Flow through any vascular bed depends on its resistance to flow and the arterial pressure. As long as this pressure is maintained constant (a critical point), alterations in flow through any individual bed will have no influence on flow through other beds in parallel with it.

A-2   (*a*) Since

$$\dot{Q} = \frac{\Delta P}{R}$$

then

$$R = \frac{\Delta P}{\dot{Q}}$$

Therefore,

$$R = \frac{100 \text{ mmHg}}{5 \text{ ml/min}}$$
$$= 20 \text{ mmHg} \cdot \text{min/ml}$$

(*b*) According to Poiseuille's equation

$$\dot{Q} = \Delta P \frac{\pi r^4}{8L} \frac{1}{\eta}$$

With other factors constant

$$\dot{Q} \; \alpha \; r^4$$

Thus doubling the radius with exercise increases flow 16-fold over that at rest. Therefore,

$$\dot{Q} = 16 \times 5 \text{ ml/min}$$
$$= 80 \text{ ml/min during exercise}$$

(c) Since

$$R = \frac{\Delta P}{\dot{Q}}$$

we have

$$R = \frac{100 \text{ mmHg}}{80 \text{ ml/min}}$$
$$= 1.25 \text{ mmHg} \cdot \text{min/ml}$$

A-3   The blood flow rate through the lungs ($\dot{Q}_L$) must equal the cardiac output (CO) because of the way the cardiovascular system is arranged. $\dot{Q}_L$ is equal to the pressure drop across the lungs (ΔP_L) divided by the resistance to flow through the lungs (R_L).

$$\text{CO} = \dot{Q}_L = \frac{\Delta P_L}{R_L} = \frac{20 \text{ mmHg}}{4 \text{ mmHg} \cdot \text{min/liter}} = 5 \text{ liters/min}$$

A-4   The Fick principle states that

$$\dot{G}_m = \dot{Q} \, ([G]_a - [G]_v)$$

Thus

$$\dot{G}_m = 60 \text{ ml/min} \times \frac{(50 - 30) \text{ mg}}{100 \text{ ml}} = 12 \text{ mg/min}$$

A-5   Since

$$\dot{F} = K[(P_c - P_i) - (\pi_c - \pi_i)]$$

then

$$\dot{F} = K[28 - (-4) - 24 + 0] \text{ mmHg} = K \times 8 \text{ mmHg}$$

The result is positive, indicating net movement of fluid *out* of the capillaries.

A-6   All do: a and d by allowing interstitial protein buildup, b by raising P_C, and c for obvious reasons.

A-7   (a) The potassium equilibrium potential will become less negative because less potential difference is required to balance the decreased tendency for net K$^+$ diffusion out of the cell. [$E_{eqK^+} = (-61.5 \text{ mV})$ log($[K^+]_i/[K^+]_o$).]
(b) Since the resting membrane is most permeable to K$^+$, the resting membrane potential is always close to the K$^+$ equilibrium potential. Lowering the absolute value of the K$^+$ equilibrium potential will undoubtedly also lower the resting membrane potential (i.e., depolarize the cells).
(c) Two things happen when the resting membrane potential is decreased: (1) the potential is closer to the threshold potential which should increase excitability and (2) the fast sodium channels become in-

activated making the cell less excitable. Thus small increases in $[K^+]_o$ may increase excitability while large increases in $[K^+]_o$ decrease excitability.

A-8 False. It is true that increases in sympathetic activity will increase heart rate (a positive chronotropic effect). However, the electrical refractory period of cardiac cells extends throughout the duration of the cell's contraction. This prevents individual twitches from ever occurring so closely together that they could summate into a tetanic state.

A-9 True. Calcium channel blockers will decrease the amount of calcium made available to the contractile machinery during excitation-contraction coupling and thus will decrease the tension-producing capabilities of the cardiac muscle cell.

A-10 a and c only. (See Figs. 3-9 and 3-10.)

A-11 The ventricular systolic pressure is also 24 mmHg since the normal pulmonic valve provides negligible resistance to flow during ejection. The right ventricular diastolic pressure, however, is determined by systemic venous pressure and will be close to 0 mmHg.

A-12 False. Although there may be minor beat-to-beat inequalities, the average stroke volumes of the right and left ventricles must be equal or blood would accumulate in the pulmonic or systemic circulation.

A-13 All of them: a by increasing preload, b by decreasing afterload, and c and d by augmenting contractility.

A-14
$$\dot{Q} = \frac{\dot{V}_{O_2}}{[O_2]_{SA} - [O_2]_{PA}}$$
$$= \frac{600 \text{ ml/min}}{(200 - 140) \text{ ml/liter}}$$
$$= 10 \text{ liters/min}$$

A-15 One cannot tell from the information given because the two alterations would have opposite effects on cardiac output. A complete set of ventricular function curves, as well as quantitative information about the changes in filling pressure and sympathetic tone, would be necessary to answer the question. (See Fig. 9-5.)

A-16 True. (See Figs. 4-6, 4-7, and, most importantly, 4-8.)

A-17 Only c.

A-18 According to the electrocardiographic conventions, the electrical axis is 90° (straight downward). Furthermore, the R wave will not appear in lead I recordings since the electrical dipole at this instant is perpendicular to the lead I axis.

A-19   a and b, because filling time is reduced; c, if ventricular rate is rapid; d, for obvious reasons; but not e, because ventricular pacemakers produce a lower heart rate, which is usually associated with a larger stroke volume.

A-20   (a) Aortic stenosis produces a significant pressure difference between the left ventricle and the aorta during systolic ejection.

(b) Mitral stenosis produces a significant pressure difference between the left atrium and the left ventricle during diastole.

A-21   Tricuspid insufficiency. With proper positioning of the patient, pulsations in the neck veins can be observed. Regurgitant flow of blood through a leaky tricuspid valve during systole produces this large abnormal c-v wave.

A-22   Irregular giant a-waves (called cannon waves) are observed in the jugular veins whenever the atrium contracts against a closed tricuspid valve (i.e., during ventricular systole). Since in third-degree heart block the atria and ventricles are beating independently, this situation may occur at irregular intervals.

A-23   True. The law of Laplace states that when the radius (r) of a cylinder increases, the wall tension (T) for a given internal pressure (P) must also increase:

$$T = P \cdot r$$

A-24   (a) By the parallel resistance equation, the equivalent resistance (R_p) for the parallel pair is $R_p = R_e/2$.
Then by the series resistance equation

$$R_n = R_e + R_p = 3R_e/2$$

(b) Since more resistance precedes the junction (R_e) than follows it ($R_e/2$), P_j will be closer to P_o than to P_i.
(c) The flow through the network (which equals the flow through the inlet vessel) is

$$\dot{Q}_n = \frac{P_i - P_o}{3R_e/2}$$

The pressure drop across the inlet vessel is equal to its resistance times the flow through it

$$P_i - P_j = R_e \frac{P_i - P_o}{3R_e/2} = 2/3(P_i - P_o)$$

A-25 Since

$$\dot{Q} = \frac{\Delta P}{R}$$

then

$$R = \frac{\Delta P}{\dot{Q}}$$

and

$$TPR = \frac{\bar{P}_A - P_{CV}}{CO}$$

Therefore

$$TPR = \frac{(100 - 0) \text{ mmHg}}{6 \text{ liters/min}}$$
$$= 16.7 \text{ mmHg} \cdot \text{min/liter}$$

A-26 False. It is less than the resistance to flow through any of the organs. Each organ, in effect, provides an additional pathway through which blood may flow; thus the individual organ resistances must be greater than the total resistance and

$$\frac{1}{TPR} = \frac{1}{R_1} + \frac{1}{R_2} + \cdots + \frac{1}{R_n}$$

A-27 False. Since

$$\frac{1}{TPR} = \frac{1}{R_{kidneys}} + \cdots$$

a decrease in renal resistance must increase 1/TPR and therefore decrease TPR. When the resistance of any single peripheral organ changes, TPR changes in the same direction.

A-28 True. Since arteriolar constriction tends to reduce the hydrostatic pressure in the capillaries, reabsorptive forces will exceed filtration forces and net reabsorption of interstitial fluid into the vascular bed will occur.

A-29 True. $\bar{P}_A = CO \times TPR$

A-30 False. Increases in cardiac output are often accompanied by decreases in total peripheral resistance. Depending on the relative magnitude of these changes, mean arterial pressure could rise, fall, or remain constant.

A-31 True. $P_p \simeq SV/C_A$. Acute changes in arterial compliance usually do not occur.

A-32 False. An increase in TRP (with CO constant) will produce approximately equal increases in P_S and P_D and increase $\bar{P}_A$ with little influence on pulse pressure.

A-33
$$\bar{P}_A \approx P_D + \tfrac{1}{3}(P_S - P_D)$$
$$\approx 70 + \tfrac{1}{3}(110 - 70) \text{ mmHg}$$
$$\approx 83 \text{ mmHg}$$

A-34   (a) Recall that $SV \simeq P_p \times C_A$. P_p increased by a factor of 1.15 (from 39 to 45 mmHg) during exercise. Since C_A is a relatively fixed parameter in the short term, the increase in P_p must have been produced by an increase in stroke volume of about 15 percent.
(b) Recall that $CO = HR \times SV$. HR increased by a factor of 2 (from 70 to 140 beats per minute) during exercise, and since SV increased by a factor of about 1.15, cardiac output must have increased by about 130 percent. [$2.0(1.15) = 2.3$ times the original level.]
(c) Recall that $TPR = \bar{P}_A/CO$. P_A increased by a factor of 1.13 (from 93 to 105 mmHg) during exercise while CO increased about 2.3 times. Thus, total peripheral resistance must have decreased by about 55 percent ($1.13/2.3 = 0.45$ of the original level.)

A-35   a, b, and c.

A-36   False. Autoregulation of blood flow implies that vascular resistance is adjusted to maintain constant flow in spite of changes in arterial pressure.

A-37   All, because they all increase myocardial oxygen consumption. Myocardial blood flow is controlled primarily by local metabolic mechanisms.

A-38   False. Sympathectomy will cause some dilation of skeletal muscle arterioles but not a maximal dilation because skeletal muscle arterioles have a strong inherent basic tone.

A-39   Hyperventilation decreases the blood P_{CO_2} level. This, in turn, causes cerebral arterioles to constrict (recall that cerebral vascular tone is highly sensitive to changes in P_{CO_2}). The increased cerebral vascular resistance causes a decrease in cerebral blood flow, which produces dizziness and disorientation.

A-40   It is likely that the increased metabolic demands evoked by the exercising skeletal muscle cannot be met by an appropriate increase in blood flow to the muscle. This patient may have some sort of arterial disease (atherosclerosis) that provides a high resistance to flow that cannot be overcome by local metabolic vasodilator mechanisms.

A-41   High left ventricular pressures must be developed to eject blood through the stenotic valve (Fig. 6-3). This increases myocardial oxygen consumption, which tends to increase coronary flow. At the same time, however, high intraventricular pressure development enhances the systolic compression of coronary vessels and tends to decrease flow. The local metabolic mechanisms may be adequate to compensate for the increased compressional forces and meet the increased myocardial metabolic needs in a resting individual. However, they may not have enough "reserve" to meet additional needs such as those that accompany exercise. Coronary perfusion pressure may also be decreased if the systemic arterial pressure is lower than normal.

A-42 Central venous pressure always settles at the value that makes cardiac output and venous return equal. Therefore anything that shifts the cardiac function curve or the venous return curve affects venous pressure (see Appendix C).

A-43 False. The Frank-Starling law says that, *if other influences on the heart are constant,* cardiac output decreases when central venous pressure decreases (e.g., A→B in Fig. 9-6). In the intact cardiovascular system, where many things may happen simultaneously, cardiac output and central venous pressure may change in opposite directions (e.g., B→C in Fig. 9-6).

A-44 None. Venous return must always equal cardiac output in the steady state situation.

A-45 a and b will increase; the rest will decrease.

A-46 Carotid sinus massage causes baroreceptors to fire, which in turn decreases sympathetic activity and increases parasympathetic activity from the medullary cardiovascular centers. Both act to slow the pacemaker activity and allows a more normal rhythm to be established.

A-47 a, b, and d increase mean arterial pressure; c and e decrease mean arterial pressure.

A-48 (1) The influence of sympathetic nerve activity on arteriolar tone will be blocked. Arteriolar tone will fall and thus so will TPR. An α blockade represents a pressure-lowering disturbance on the effector portion of the cardiovascular system.
(2) The effector portion function curve will shift downward as shown in Fig. 10-6B (In this instance the effector function curve may also become less steep, because increases in TPR no longer aid in the production of increased P_A when sympathetic activity increases.)
(3) A new steady state will be established within the arterial baroreceptor reflex pathway at lower than normal arterial pressure and higher than normal sympathetic nerve activity, as shown in Fig. 10-6B.
(4) Heart rate and cardiac output will increase because of the increased sympathetic activity. The cardiac function curve will shift upward, but the venous return curve will not because alpha-receptor blockade blocks the effect of increased sympathetic activity on the veins. Consequently, central venous pressure will be lower than normal (see Fig. 9-5).

A-49 a and d are disturbances to the effector portion of the arterial baroreceptor control system which reduce the arterial pressure produced for any given level of sympathetic activity. Thus, as indicated in Fig. 10-6*B*, the net results of these disturbances and subsequent adjustments to them will be a new steady state at a lower than normal mean arterial pressure and a higher than normal sympathetic activity.

b and c elicit set-point-increasing inputs to the neural portion of the arterial baroreceptor control system that result in a greater than normal sympathetic output for any given level of input from the arterial baroreceptors. Thus, as indicated in Fig. 10-7*A*, in the presence of these disturbances the system will operate at higher than normal mean arterial pressure and sympathetic activity.

A-50 a and c. These disturbances would tend to directly lower blood pressure which would then lead to a reflex increase in heart rate. Disturbances b and d have no direct effect on the heart or vessels. Rather they act on the medullary cardiovascular centers to raise the set point and cause an increase in sympathetic activity. Consequently, one would expect b and d to cause increases in *both* heart rate and mean arterial pressure.

A-51 Because capillaries have such a small radius, the tension in the capillary wall is rather modest despite very high internal pressures ($T = P \cdot r$).

A-52 Fainting occurs because of decreased cerebral blood flow when mean arterial pressure falls below about 60 mmHg. On a hot day, temperature reflexes override pressure reflexes to produce the increased skin blood flow required for thermal regulation. Thus TPR is lower when standing on a hot day than on a cool one. Consequently, mean arterial pressure falls below 60 mmHg with less lowering of cardiac output on a warm day than on a cool one.

A-53 The cardiovascular response to lying down is just the opposite of that shown in Fig. 11-3. Patients tend to lose rather than retain fluid during extended bed rest and end up with lower than normal blood volumes. Thus they are less able to cope with an upright posture during the period required for blood volume to reachieve the value it has when periods of standing are part of the patient's normal routine.

A-54 The pressure produced by the water on the lower part of the body enhances reabsorption of fluid into the capillaries, reduces the peripheral venous volume, and increases the volume of blood in the central venous pool. This stimulates the cardiopulmonary mechanoreceptors and evokes a diuresis by way of the various neural and hormonal pathways discussed in Chap. 10.

A-55 $R = \bar{P}_A/\dot{Q}$. Skeletal muscle resistance must have decreased considerably during exercise because skeletal muscle flow increased 10-fold (1000 percent) whereas mean arterial pressure increased much less ($\simeq$ 11 percent).

A-56 TPR $= \bar{P}_A/CO$. Total peripheral resistance must have decreased during exercise because cardiac output increased threefold, which is relatively much larger than the increase in mean arterial pressure.

A-57 (1) The heart rate during exercise is well above the intrinsic rate ($\simeq 100$ beats per minute). This indicates activation of the cardiac sympathetic nerves because withdrawal of cardiac parasympathetic activity cannot increase heart rate above the intrinsic rate (Chap. 3).
(2) Increased arterial pulse pressure at constant central venous pressure indicates increased stroke volume and cardiac contractility and thus increased activity of cardiac sympathetic nerves (Chap. 4).
(3) Decreased renal and splanchnic blood flows in spite of increased mean arterial pressure indicate sympathetic vasoconstriction (Chap. 5).

A-58 (a)   SV = CO/HR
SV $= 6,000/70 = 86$ ml/beat at rest.
SV $= 18,000/160 = 113$ ml/beat during exercise.

[You may recall that, in the absence of other information, changes in *SV* can be *estimated* from changes in arterial pulse pressure, (P_p). The information in Fig. 11-4 indicates that P_p increased 1.75-times (from 40 mmHg to 70 mmHg) as a result of exercise whereas *SV* actually increased only 1.32-times (from 86 ml to 113 ml), as calculated earlier. This discrepancy emphasizes that while *SV* is a major determinant of P_p, changes in other factors, such as the compliance of arteries (C_A), can influence P_p as well (see Appendix C). Part of the increase in P_p that accompanies exercise is due to a *decrease* in effective arterial compliance. The latter is due to (1) an increase in mean arterial pressure with exercise, and (2) the nonlinear nature of the arterial volume-pressure relationship (see Fig. 7-10).]
(b) Ejection fraction = SV/EDV, or EDV = SV/ejection fraction

EDV $= 86/0.60 = 143$ ml at rest
EDV $= 113/0.80 = 141$ ml during exercise

[Recall that central venous pressure, P_{CV}, is the cardiac filling pressure or preload and is therefore the primary determinant of EDV. The EDV changed little with exercise because exercise caused little or no change in P_{CV}.]
(c) SV = EDV − ESV, or ESV = EDV − SV

ESV $= 143 - 86 = 57$ ml at rest
ESV $= 141 - 113 = 28$ ml during exercise

[Recall that the primary determinants of ESV are cardiac afterload (mean arterial pressure) and myocardial contractility (see Appendix C). Cardiac afterload increases during exercise and thus goes in the wrong direction to account for a decrease in ESV. Therefore, an increased myocardial contractility, secondary to increased cardiac sympathetic nerve activity, must be primarily responsible for the decrease in ESV that accompanies exercise.]

(d)

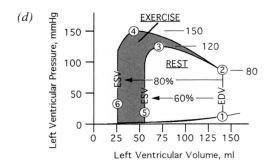

Left Ventricular Volume, ml

Key features:

1 End-diastolic volume during both rest and exercise is about 140 ml.
2 Ventricular ejection (decreasing ventricular volume) begins when intraventricular pressure reaches the diastolic aortic pressure and the aortic valve opens. Figure 11-4 indicates an arterial diastolic pressure of 80 mmHg both at rest and during exercise. Thus, ventricular ejection will begin at an intraventricular pressure of 80 mmHg in both situations.
3 and **4** Peak intraventricular pressure normally equals peak (systolic) arterial pressure. Hence, the systolic arterial pressure values in Fig. 11-4 indicate peak intraventricular pressures of 120 mmHg and 150 mmHg during rest and exercise, respectively.
5 and **6** As calculated in c earlier, end-systolic volume is 57 ml at rest and decreases to 28 ml during exercise.

A-59 When the lungs are inflated artificially, intrathoracic pressure goes up (rather than down, as occurs during normal inspiration). On the average, intrathoracic pressure and thus central venous pressure are higher than normal with artificial respiration. In this situation, however, higher than normal central venous pressure does not increase cardiac filling significantly because a parallel increase in pressure occurs on the outside of the heart. The increased central venous pressure does inhibit venous return, and this is what causes the adverse cardiovascular effects of positive pressure respiration.

A-60 Blood flow through muscle is reduced or stopped by compressive forces on skeletal muscle vessels during an isometric muscle contraction. Thus, during an isometric maneuver, TPR may be higher than normal rather than much lower than normal as it is during phasic exercises such as running. In the absence of decreased TPR but the presence of strong set-point-raising influences (central command) from the cortex on the medullary cardiovascular centers, mean arterial pressure may be regulated to very high values (see point 2 in Fig. 10-6A).

A-61 Intense sympathetic activation drastically reduces skin blood flow, promotes transcapillary reabsorption of fluids, increases heart rate and contractility (but may not restore stroke volume because of low central venous pressure), and reduces skeletal muscle blood flow. Cerebral blood flow falls if the compensatory mechanisms do not prevent mean arterial pressure from falling below 60 mmHg.

A-62 (*a*) Not helpful since gravity tends to promote peripheral venous blood pooling and cause a further fall in arterial pressure.
(*b*) Not helpful if carried to an extreme. Cutaneous vasodilation produced by warming adds to the cardiovascular stresses.
(*c*) Helpful if the victim is conscious and can drink since fluid will be rapidly absorbed from the gut to increase circulating blood volume.
(*d*) Might be helpful as an initial emergency measure to prevent brain damage due to severely reduced blood pressure, but prolonged treatment will promote the decompensatory mechanisms associated with decreased organ blood flow.

A-63 (*a*) In hypovolemic shock from diarrhea, the hematocrit will probably increase because, even though the compensatory processes will evoke a substantial "auto transfusion" by shifting fluid from the intracellular and interstitial space into the vascular space, this amount of fluid is limited to a liter or less. Therefore, a substantial loss of fluid (without red blood cells) will *raise* the hematocrit significantly.
(*b*) In cardiogenic shock, the hematocrit may decrease because compensatory actions evoked to maintain blood pressure may promote a fluid shift into the vascular space. However, since central venous pressure (and perhaps peripheral venous pressures) may also be elevated, capillary hydrostatic pressures (and thus fluid shifts) are difficult to predict.
(*c*) In septic shock, peripheral vasodilation and peripheral venous pooling may actually promote filtration of fluid out of the vasculature in some beds (which would lead to an increased hematocrit) but the low arterial and central venous pressures may counteract this shift so changes in hematocrits are difficult to predict in this situation.
(*d*) Chronic bleeding disorders are usually associated with low hematocrit and anemia because red blood cell production may not keep pace with red cell losses whereas the volume regulating mechanisms may be able to maintain a normal blood volume.

A-64 Excessive fluid retention can induce decompensatory mechanisms that further compromise an already weakened heart (e.g., inadequate oxygenation of the blood as it passes through edematous lungs, marked cardiac dilation and increased myocardial metabolic needs, liver dysfunction due to congestion). Diuretic therapy reduces fluid volume and the high venous pressures that are the cause of these problems.

A-65 If blood volume and central venous pressure are reduced too far with diuretic therapy, cardiac output may fall to unacceptably low levels through the Frank-Starling law.

A-66 Because of the high resistance of the stenosis and the pressure drop across it, glomerular capillary pressure and therefore glomerular filtration rate are lower than normal when arterial pressure is normal. Thus a renal artery stenosis reduces the urine output rate caused by a given level of arterial pressure. The renal function curve is shifted to the right, and hypertension follows.

SUGGESTED READINGS

GENERAL

To keep abreast of continuing developments in cardiovascular physiology, interested students should peruse the following journals: *American Journal of Physiology: Heart and Circulatory Physiology, Circulation Research, Journal of Molecular and Cellular Cardiology, and Microvascular Research.* Excellent detailed review articles on cardiovascular physiology are periodically published in *News in Physiological Sciences, Annual Reviews of Physiology, Physiological Reviews,* and *Circulation Research.* In addition, *Circulation, New England Journal of Medicine,* and *Progress in Cardiovascular Diseases* often contain review articles which emphasize the clinical applications of recent cardiovascular research findings.

CHAP. 1

Aukland K and RK Reed: Interstitial-lymphatic mechanisms in the control of extracellular volume. *Physiol Rev,* vol 73, 1993, pp 1–78.

Chien S, S Usami, and R Skalak: Blood flow in small tubes. *Handbook of Physiology,* 2nd ed, sec 2, vol 4, ed by EM Renkin and CC Michel, American Physiological Society, Bethesda, 1984, pp 217–250.

Clough G: Relationship between microvascular permeability and ultrastructure. *Progress in Biophysics and Molecular Biology,* vol 55, 1991, pp 47–69.

Crone C and DG Levitt: Capillary permeability to small solutes. *Handbook of Physiology,* 2nd ed, sec 2, vol 4, ed by EM Renkin and CC Michel, American Physiological Society, Bethesda, 1984. pp 411–466.

Curry FE: Mechanics and thermodynamics of transcapillary exchange. *Handbook of Physiology,* 2nd ed, sec 2, vol 4, ed by EM Renkin and CC Michel, American Physiological Society, Bethesda, 1984, pp 309–374.

Curry FE: Regulation of water and solute exchange in microvessel endothelium: Studies in single perfused capillaries. *Microcirculation,* vol 1, 1994, pp 11–26.

Michel CC: Fluid movements through capillary walls. *Handbook of Physiology,* 2nd ed, sec 2, vol 4, ed by EM Renkin and CC Michel, American Physiological Society, Bethesda, 1984, pp 375–410.

Parker JC, MA Perry, and AE Taylor: Permeability of the microvascular barrier. *Edema.* NC Staub and AE Taylor (eds). Raven Press, New York, 1984, pp 143–187.

Predescu D and GE Palade: Plasmalemmal vesicles represent the large pore system of continuous microvascular endothelium. *Amer J Physiol,* vol 265(2 pt 2), 1993, pp H725–H733.

Renkin EM and CC Michel (eds): *Handbook of Physiology,* sec 2: The Cardiovascular System, vol 4: Microcirculation. American Physiological Society, Bethesda, 1984.

Renkin EM and VL Tucker: Atrial natriuretic peptide as a regulator of transvascular fluid balance. *NIPS,* vol 11, 1996, pp 138–143.

Rippe B and B Haraldsson: Transport of macromolecules across microvascular walls: The two-pore theory. *Physiol Rev,* vol 74, 1994, pp 163–219.

Schmid-Schonbein GW and BW Zweifach: Fluid pump mechanisms in initial lymphatics. *NIPS,* vol 9, 1994, pp 67–71.

Starling EH: On the absorption of fluids from the connective tissue spaces. *J Physiol (London),* vol 19, 1896, p 312.

Taylor AE and DN Granger: Exchange of macromolecules across the microcirculation. *Handbook of Physiology,* 2nd ed, sec 2, vol 4, ed by EM Renkin and CC Michel, American Physiological Society, Bethesda, 1984, pp 467–520.

Wagner RC and SC Chen: Transcapillary transport of solute by the endothelial vesicular system: Evidence from thin serial section analysis. *Microvascular Res,* vol 42, 1991, pp 139–150.

Zweifach BW and A Silberberg: The interstitial-lymphatic flow system. *Int Rev Physiol Cardiovasc Physiol III,* vol 18, 1979, pp 215–260.

Zweifach BW and HH Lipowsky: Pressure-flow relations in blood and lymph microcirculation. *Handbook of Physiology,* 2nd ed, sec 2, vol 4, ed by EM Renkin and CC Michel, American Physiological Society, Bethesda, 1984, pp 251–308.

CHAPS. 2–6

Billman GE: Cellular mechanisms for ventricular fibrillation. *NIPS,* vol 7, 1992, pp 254–259.

Brady AJ: Mechanical properties of isolated cardiac myocytes. *Physiol Rev,* vol 71, 1991, pp 413–422.

Catterall WA: Cellular and molecular biology of voltage-gated sodium channels. *Physiol Rev,* vol 72 (Suppl), 1992, S15–S48.

Coraboeuf E and D Escande: Ionic currents in the human myocardium. *NIPS,* vol 5, 1990, pp 28–31.

DiFrancesco D: Pacemaker mechanisms in cardiac tissue. *Ann Rev Physiol,* vol 55, 1993, pp 451–467.

Elzinga G: Starling's "law of the heart": Rise and fall of the descending limb. *NIPS,* vol 7, 1992, pp 134–137.

Fuchs F: Mechanical modulation of the Ca^{2+} regulatory protein complex in cardiac muscle. *NIPS,* vol 10, 1995, pp 6–12.

Hirst GDS, FR Edwards, NJ Bramich, and MF Klemm: Neural control of cardiac pacemaker potentials. *NIPS,* vol 6, 1991, pp 185–190.

Howell WH and F Donaldson: Experiments upon the heart of the dog with reference to the maximum volume of blood sent out by the left ventricle in a single beat and the influence of variations in venous pressure, arterial pressure and pulse rate upon the work done by the heart. *Philos Trans R Soc London,* vol 175, pt 1, 1884, pp 139–160.

Irisawa H, HF Brown, and W Giles: Cardiac pacemaking in the sinoatrial node. *Physiol Rev,* vol 73, 1993, pp 197–227.

Jongsma HJ and D Gros: The cardiac connection. *NIPS,* vol 6, 1991, pp 34–40.

Katz AM: *Physiology of the Heart,* 2nd ed. Raven Press, New York, 1992.

Langer GA: Calcium and the heart: exchange at the tissue, cell and organelle levels. *FASEB Journal,* vol 6, 1992, pp 893–902.

McDonald TF, S Pelzer, W Trautwein, and DJ Pelzer: Regulation and modulation of calcium channels in cardiac skeletal, and smooth muscle cells. *Physiol Rev,* vol 74, 1994, pp 365–507.

Noble D: The surprising heart: A review of recent progress in cardiac electrophysiology. *J Physiol,* vol 353, 1984, pp 1–50.

Obeid AI: *Electrophysiology in Clinical Practice.* JB Lippincott, Philadelphia, 1992.

Pallotta BS and PK Wagoner: Voltage-dependent potassium channels since Hodgkin and Huxley. *Physiol Rev,* vol 72 (Suppl), 1992, pp S49–S67.

Pongs O: Molecular biology of voltage-dependent potassium channels. *Physiol Rev,* vol 72(Suppl), 1992, S69–S88.

Rosenshtraukh LV and AV Zaitsev: Atrial tachycardias—A new look. *NIPS,* vol 5, 1990, pp 187–190.

Sagawa K: The end-systolic pressure-volume relationship of the ventricles: Definition, modification and clinical use. *Circulation,* vol 63, 1981, pp 1223–1227.

Sarnoff SJ: Myocardial contractility as described by ventricular function curves. *Physiol Rev,* vol 35, 1955, p 107.

Saul JP: Beat-to-beat variations of heart rate reflect modulation of cardiac autonomic outflow. *NIPS,* vol 5, 1990, pp 32–37.

Starling EH: *The Linacre Lecture on the Law of the Heart.* Longmans Green, London, 1918.

Zipes DP and J Jalife: *Cardiac Electrophysiology: From Cell to Bedside.* Saunders, Philadelphia, 1990.

CHAPS. 7–8

Bevan JA and RD Bevan: Is innervation a prime regulator of cerebral blood flow? *NIPS,* vol 8, 1993, pp 149–152.

Bohr DF, AP Somlyo, and HV Sparks Jr (eds): *Handbook of Physiology,* sec 2: The Cardiovascular System, vol 2: *Vascular Smooth Muscle.* Bethesda, American Physiological Society, 1980, Chaps. 4, 12, 13, 15–20.

Bradbury MWB: The blood-brain barrier. *Experimental Physiol,* vol 78, 1993, 453–472.

Brown AM: Ion channels as G protein effectors. *NIPS,* vol 6, 1991, pp 158–161.

Brutsaert DL: Endocardial and coronary endothelial control of cardiac performance. *NIPS,* vol 8, 1993, pp 82–86.

Calver A, J Collier, and P Vallance: Nitric oxide and cardiovascular control. *Experimental Physiol,* vol 78, 1993, pp 303–326.

Chien S, S Usami, and R Skalak: Blood flow in small tubes. *Handbook of Physiology,* 2nd ed, sec 2, vol 4, ed by EM Renkin and CC Michel, American Physiological Society, Bethesda, 1984, pp 217–250.

Ellsworth ML, CG Ellis, AS Popel, and RN Pittman: Role of microvessels in oxygen supply to tissue. *NIPS,* vol 9, 1994, pp 119–123.

Gerova M: Conduit coronary artery: Control by autonomic nervous system. *NIPS,* vol 6, 1991, pp 103–107.

Gewirtz H: The coronary circulation: Limitations of current concepts of metabolic control. *NIPS,* vol 6, 1991, pp 265–268.

Gorman MW and HV Sparks: The unanswered question. (What is the dilator substance in exercise hyperemia?). *NIPS,* vol 6, 1991, pp 191–193.

Hainsworth R: The importance of vascular capacitance in cardiovascular control. *NIPS,* vol 5, 1990, pp 250–254.

Hirst GD and FR Edwards: Sympathetic neuroeffector transmission in arteries and arterioles. *Physiol Rev,* vol 69, 1989, pp 546–604.

Johnson PC: Autoregulation of blood flow. *Circ Res,* vol 59, 1986, pp 483–495.

Johnson PC: The myogenic response. *NIPS,* vol 6, 1991, pp 41–42.

Kamm KE and JT Stull: Regulation of smooth muscle contractile elements by second messengers. *Ann Rev Physiol,* vol 51, 1989, pp 299–313.

Mellander S and J Bjornberg: Regulation of vascular smooth muscle tone and capillary pressure. *NIPS,* vol 7, 1992, pp 113–119.

Murphy RA: Special topic: Contraction in smooth muscle cells. *Ann Rev Physiol,* vol 51, 1989, pp 275–349.

O'Donnell ME and NE Owen: Regulation of ion pumps and carriers in vascular smooth muscle. *Physiol Rev,* vol 74, 1994, pp 683–721.

Rhodin JAG: Architecture of the vessel wall, in *Handbook of Physiology,* sec 2: The Cardiovascular System, vol 2: *Vascular Smooth Muscle,* ed by DF Bohr, AP Somlyo, and HV Sparks Jr. Bethesda, American Physiological Society, 1980.

Robinshaw D and KA Foster: Role of G proteins in the regulation of the cardiovascular system. *Ann Rev Physiol,* vol 51, 1989, pp 229–244.

Rowell LB: The venous system, in *Human Circulation: Regulation During Physical Stress.* Oxford University Press, New York, 1986, pp 44–77.

Smiesko V and PC Johnson: The arterial lumen is controlled by flow-related shear stress. *NIPS,* vol 8, 1993, pp 34–38.

Suzuki H and G Chen: Endothelium-derived hyperpolarizing factor (EDHF): An endogenous potassium-channel activator. *NIPS,* vol 5, 1990, pp 212–215.

West JB and O Mathieu-Costello: Pulmonary blood-gas barrier: A physiological dilemma. *NIPS,* vol 8, 1993, pp 249–253.

CHAPS. 9–10

Anderson MC and DL Kunze: Nucleus tractus solitarius—gateway to neural circulatory control. *Ann Rev Physiol,* vol 56, 1994, pp 93–116.

Blessing WW: Inhibitory vasomotor neurons in the caudal ventrolateral medulla oblongata. *NIPS,* vol 6, 1991, pp 139–141.

Calaresu FR and CP Yardley: Medullary basal sympathetic tone. *Ann Rev Physiol,* vol 50, 1988, pp 511–524.

Chapleau MW, G Hajduczok, and FM Abboud: Paracrine modulation of baroreceptor activity by vascular endothelium. *NIPS,* vol 6, 1991, pp 210–214.

Cowley AW, Jr: Long-term control of arterial blood pressure. *Physiol Rev,* vol 72, 1992, pp 231–300.

Cushing H: Concerning a definite regulatory mechanism of the vasomotor center which controls blood pressure during cerebral compression. *Bull Johns Hopkins Hosp,* vol 12, 1901, pp 290.

Dampney R: The subretrofacial nucleus: Its pivotal role in cardiovascular regulation. *NIPS,* vol 5, 1990, pp 63–67.

Dampney RA: Functional organization of central pathways regulating the cardiovascular system. *Physiol Rev,* vol 74, 1994, pp 323–364.

Eckberg DL and JM Fritsch: How should human baroreflexes be tested? *NIPS,* vol 8, 1993, pp 7–12.

Eckberg DL and P Sleight. *Human Baroreflexes in Health and Disease.* Clarendon Press, Oxford, 1992.

Gorman MW and HV Sparks: The unanswered question (What is the dilator substance in exercise hyperemia?). *NIPS,* vol 6, 1991, pp 191–193.

Guyton AC: Determination of cardiac output by equating venous return curves with cardiac response curves. *Physiol Rev,* vol 35, 1955, pp 123.

Hainsworth R: Reflexes from the heart. *Physiol Rev,* vol 71, 1991, pp 617–658.

Lakatta EG: Cardiovascular regulatory mechanisms in advanced age. *Physiol Rev,* vol 73, 1993, pp 413–460.

Longhurst JC: Cardiopulmonary receptors: Their function in health and disease. *Prog Cardiovasc Diseases,* vol 27(3), 1984, pp 201–222.

Marshall JM: Peripheral chemoreceptors and cardiovascular regulation. *Physiol Rev,* vol 74, 1994, pp 543–594.

Paton JFR and KM Spyer: Cerebellar cortical regulation of circulation. *NIPS,* vol 7, 1992, pp 124–129.

Rothe CF: Mean circulatory filling pressure: its meaning and measurement. *J Applied Physiology,* vol 74, 1993, pp 499–509.

Rowell LB: Cardiovascular aspects of human temperature regulation. *Circ Res,* vol 52, 1983, pp 367–379.

Rowell LB: *Human Cardiovascular Control,* Oxford University Press, New York, 1993.

Sarnoff SJ: Myocardial contractility as described by cardiac function curves. *Physiol Rev,* vol 35, 1955, pp 107.

Segal SS: Communication among endothelial and smooth muscle cells coordinates blood flow control during exercise. *NIPS,* vol 7, 1992, pp 152–156.

Shepherd JT, and FM Abboud (eds): *Handbook of Physiology,* sec. 2: The Cardiovascular System, vol 3: *Peripheral Circulation and Organ Blood Flow,* American Physiology Society, Bethesda, 1983, Chaps 15, 19–21.

Spyer KM: Central nervous system mechanisms contributing to cardiovascular control. *J Physiol,* vol 474, 1994, pp 1–19.

Starling EH: *The Linacre Lecture on the Law of the Heart.* Longmans Green, London, 1918.

Vander AJ: *Renal Physiology,* 5th ed, McGraw-Hill, New York, 1995.

Williams JL, KL Barnes, BK Brosnihan, and CM Farrario: Area postrema: A unique regulator of cardiovascular function, *NIPS,* vol 7, 1992, pp 30–34.

CHAPS. 11–12

Aukland K: Why don't our feet swell in the upright position? *NIPS,* vol 9, 1994, pp 214–219.

Blomqvist CG and HL Stone: Cardiovascular adjustments to gravitational stress, in *Handbook of Physiology,* sec 2: The Cardiovascular System, vol 3: *Peripheral Circulation and Organ Blood Flow,* ed. by JT Shepherd and FM Abboud, American Physiological Society, Bethesda, 1983, pp 1025–1063.

Cruickshank JM and BNC Prichard: *Beta-Blockers in Clinical Practice.* Churchill Livingstone, New York, 1994.

Dietz HC III and RE Pyeritz. Molecular genetic approaches to the study of cardiovascular disease. *Ann Rev Physiol,* vol 56, 1994, pp 763–796.

DiNicolantonio R, T Imai, K Murakami, and Y Yamori: Hypertension: Genes, environment, or both? *NIPS,* vol 6, 1991, pp 174–177.

Dominiczak A, and K Lindpaintner: Genetics of hypertension: A current appraisal. *NIPS,* vol 9, 1994, pp 246–251.

Folkow B: Salt and hypertension. *NIPS,* vol 5, 1990, pp 220–224.

Folkow B and A Svanborg: Physiology of cardiovascular aging. *Physiol Rev,* vol 73, 1993, pp 725–764.

Francis GS and JN Cohn: Heart failure: Mechanisms of cardiac and vascular dysfunction and the rationale for pharmacologic intervention. *FASEB Journal,* vol 4, 1990, pp 3068–3075.

Garcia R: Atrial natriuretic factor in experimental and human hypertension. *NIPS,* vol 8, 1993, pp 161–164.

Goldstein DS: *Stress, Catecholamines, and Cardiovascular Disease.* Oxford University Press, New York, 1995.

Haddy FJ: Humoral factors in hypertension. *NIPS,* vol 4, 1989, pp 202–205.

Homy CJ, SF Vatner, and DE Vatner: β-adrenergic receptor regulation in the heart in pathophysiological states: Abnormal adrenergic responsiveness in cardiac disease. *Ann Rev Physiol,* vol 53, 1991, pp 137–159.

Kedes L: Regulation of myocardial adaptation. *Scientific Amer Sci Med,* July/August, 1994.

Kovach AGB and AM Lefer: Endothelial dysfunction in shock states. *NIPS,* vol 8, 1993, pp 145–148.

Lahera V and AA Khraibi: Nitric oxide inhibition in hypertension. *NIPS,* vol 9, 1994, pp 268–170.

Ludbrook J and R Evans: Posthemorrhagic syncope. *NIPS,* vol 4, 1989, pp 120–133.

Luscher TF and Y Dohi: Endothelium-derived relaxing factor and endothelin in hypertension. *NIPS,* vol 7, 1992, pp 120–123.

Navas JP and M Martinez-Maldonado: Pathophysiology of edema in congestive heart failure. *Heart Dis & Stroke,* vol 2, 1993, pp 325–329.

Opie LH: ACE inhibitors: almost too good to be true. *Sci Amer Sci Med,* July/Aug 1994.

Winaver J, A Hoffman, Z Abassi, and A Haramati: Does the heart's hormone, ANP, help in congestive heart failure? *NIPS,* vol 10, 1995, pp 247–253.

Zucker IH, W Wang and M Brandle: Baroreflex abnormalities in congestive heart failure. *NIPS,* vol 8, 1993, pp 87–90.

APPENDICES

APPENDIX A

Normal Values of Erythrocytes, Leukocytes and Platelets in Human Blood

Erythrocytes		5,000,000 per mm^3 of blood	
Platelets		250,000 per mm^3 of blood	
Leukocytes		7000 per mm^3 of blood	
Type of leukocyte	Percent total leukocytes	Primary role
Polymorphonuclear Granulocytes		
Neutrophils	50–70	Phagocytosis
Eosinophils	1–4	Allergic hypersensitivity reactions
Basophils	0–0.75	Allergic hypersensitivity reactions
Monocytes	2–8	Phagocytosis and antibody production
Lymphocytes	20–40	Antibody production and cell-mediated immunity

APPENDIX B

Normal Constituents of Adult Human Plasma

Class	Constituent	Amount/ normal concentration range
Electrolytes (inorganic)		
Cations	Sodium (Na$^+$)	136–145 mEq/L
	Potassium (K$^+$)	3.5–5.0 mEq/L
	Calcium (Ca^{2+})	4.3–5.2 mEq/L
	Magnesium (Mg^{2+})	1.2–1.8 mEq/L
	Iron (Fe^{3+})	60–160 μg/dl
	Copper (Cu^{2+})	70–155 μg/dl
	Hydrogen (H$^+$)	35–45 nmol/L (pH = 7.35–7.45)
Anions	Chloride (Cl$^-$)	98–106 mEq/L
	Bicarbonate (HCO$_3^-$)	23–28 mEq/L
	Lactate	0.67–1.8 mEq/L
	Sulfate (SO$_4^{2-}$)	0.9–1.1 mEq/L
	Phosphate (HPO$_4^{2-}$mostly)	3.0–4.5 mg/dl
Proteins	Total (7% of plasma weight)	6–8 g/dl
	Albumin	3.4–5.0 g/dl
	Globulins	2.2–4.0 g/dl
	Fibrinogen	0.3 g/dl
Nutrients	Glucose	80–120 mg/dl
	Total amino acids	40 mg/dl
	Cholesterol	150–200 mg/dl
	Phospholipids	150–220 mg/dl
	Triglycerides	35–160 mg/dl
Waste products	Uric acid (from nucleic acids)	2.6–7.2 mg/dl
	Blood urea nitrogen (from protein)	8–25 mg/dl
	Creatinine (from creatine)	0.2–0.9 mg/dl
	Bilirubin (from heme)	0.1–1.2 mg/dl

APPENDIX C

Key Cardiovascular Variables and Their Normal Determinants[1]

$$\bar{P}_A = CO \times TPR$$

$$CO = SV \times HR$$

$$SV = EDV - ESV$$

$$ejection\ fraction = SV/EDV$$

$SV \xleftarrow{\text{ventricular pump}}$
- $(+) \uparrow$ cardiac preload (via effect on EDV)
- $(+) \uparrow$ cardiac contractility (via effect on ESV)
- $(-) \uparrow$ cardiac afterload (via effect on ESV)

$$cardiac\ preload \propto P_{CV} \qquad (\text{``}\propto\text{'' means ``is proportional to''})$$

$P_{CV} \xleftarrow{\text{central blood volume}}$
- $(+) \uparrow$ total blood volume
- $(+) \uparrow$ peripheral venous tone
- $(+)$ skeletal muscle pump
- $(+)$ respiratory pump
- $(-)$ standing
- $(-) \uparrow$ cardiac output

$venous\ tone \xleftarrow{\hspace{2cm}} \{(+) \uparrow$ sympathetic activity, (via NE, α-receptors)

$contractility \xleftarrow{\text{ventricular cells}} \{(+) \uparrow$ sympathetic activity, (via NE, β-receptors)

$$cardiac\ afterload \propto \bar{P}_A$$

$HR \xleftarrow{\text{SA node cell firing rate}}$
- $(+) \uparrow$ sympathetic activity, (via NE, β-receptors)
- $(-) \uparrow$ parasympathetic activity, (via ACh)

$TPR \xleftarrow{\text{arteriolar tone}}$
- $(+) \uparrow$ sympathetic activity, (via NE, α-receptors)
- $(-) \uparrow$ local metabolites, ($\uparrow$ local metabolic rate)

$$P_P \propto SV/C_A$$

$C_A \xleftarrow{\text{large artery elasticity}} \{(-) \uparrow$ age

---

1 P_A, mean arterial pressure; CO, cardiac output; TPR, total peripheral resistance; SV, stroke volume; HR, heart rate; ESV, end-systolic volume; EDV, end-diastolic volume; P_{CV}, central venous pressure; NE, norepinephrine; ACh, acetylcholine; P_P, arterial pulse pressure; C_A, arterial compliance; SA, sinoatrial.

APPENDIX D
Hemostasis

Whenever damage occurs to a blood vessel, a variety of processes are evoked that are aimed at preventing or stopping blood from exiting the vascular space. The three primary processes are summarized in the following list:

I   Platelet Aggregation and Plug Formation: occurs as a result of the following steps:
  A   Vessel injury with endothelial damage and collagen exposure.
  B   Platelet adherence to collagen (mediated by the plasma protein, von Willebrand factor).
  C   Platelet shape change (from discs to spiny spheres) and degranulation with release of the following:
    1   Adenosine diphosphate, which causes platelet aggregation and "plugs" the hole.
    2   Thromboxane, which causes vasoconstriction and potentiates platelet adhesion and aggregation.

(Aspirin and other cyclooxygenase inhibitors are anticoagulants because they prevent the formation of thromboxane.)

II   Local Vasoconstriction: mediated largely by thromboxane, but also may be induced by local release of other chemical signals that constrict local vessels and reduce blood flow.
III   Blood Clotting: the formation of a solid gel made up of the protein, fibrin, platelets, and trapped blood cells.

The critical step in blood clotting is the formation of thrombin from prothrombin, which then catalyzes the conversion of fibrinogen to fibrin. The final clot is stabilized by covalent cross-linkages between fibrin strands catalyzed by factor XIIIa (the formation of which is catalyzed by thrombin).

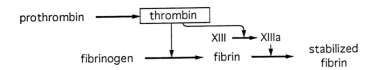

The cascade of reactions that leads from vessel injury to the formation of thrombin is shown in the succeeding figure and is described as follows:

  A   Vessel injury with blood exposure to subendothelial cells with "tissue factor" on their cell membranes.
  B   The plasma protein, factor VII, binds to the tissue factor which converts it to an activated form, factor VIIa.
  C   VIIa catalyzes conversion of both factors IX and X to activated forms, IXa and Xa, respectively.

D IXa also helps convert factor X to Xa (Stuart factor).

E Xa converts prothrombin to thrombin.

F Thrombin

    1 Activates platelets (makes them sticky, induces degranulation, promotes attachment of various factors that participate in clotting).

    2 Converts fibrinogen to fibrin.

    3 Recruits the "intrinsic pathway," which amplifies further formation of factor Xa and facilitates the conversion of prothrombin to thrombin by promoting the following reactions:

        a Conversion of factor XI to its activated form, XIa, which then converts factor IX to IXa, which then attaches to activated platelets and converts factor X to Xa.

        b Conversion of factor VIII (missing in hemophiliacs) to its activated form, VIIIa, which attaches to activated platelets and accelerates conversion of factor X to Xa.

        c Conversion of factor V to its activated form, Va, which attaches to activated platelets and accelerates conversion of prothrombin to thrombin.

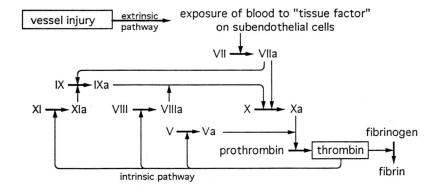

(Several agents clinically used as *anticoagulants* interfere with various steps in this clotting process. *Dicoumarol* and *coumadin* block the activity of vitamin K, which is necessary for synthesis of many of the clotting factors by the liver. *Heparin* activates a plasma protein called antithrombin III which, in turn, inactivates thrombin and several of the other clotting factors. Because calcium is an important clotting cofactor, calcium chelators such as *EDTA, oxalate,* and *citrate* are used to prevent stored blood from clotting. Various *thrombolytic agents* modeled after the endogenous *tissue plasminogen activator (tPA)* are also available that promote dissolution of the fibrin clot after it is formed. These agents promote the formation of plasmin from plasminogen which enzymatically attacks the clot turning it into soluble peptides.)

INDEX

Page numbers in *italics* refer to illustrations;
those ending in the letter *t* refer to tables.